Adult Aphasia Rehabilitation

Adult Aphasia Rehabilitation: Applied Pragmatics

G. Albyn Davis, Ph.D.
University of Massachusetts at Amherst
and
M. Jeanne Wilcox, Ph.D.
Kent State University

COLLEGE-HILL PRESS, San Diego, California

College-Hill Press, Inc.
4284 41st Street
San Diego, California 92105

Library of Congress Cataloging in Publication Data
Main entry under title:

Davis, G. Albyn (George Albyn), 1946–
    Adult aphasia rehabilitation.

    Includes bibliographies and index. 1. Aphasics—Rehabilitation. 2. Speech
therapy. I. Wilcox, M. Jeanne, 1953–   . II. Title. [DNLM: 1. Aphasia—in
adulthood. 2. Aphasia—rehabilitation. 3. Speech Therapy—methods. WL 340.5
D261a]
RC425.D378   1985   616.85′5206   85–6679

ISBN 0–88744–195–5 (pbk.)

Printed in the United States of America

CONTENTS

PREFACE

Our main purpose in writing this book is to introduce the speech-language pathologist to the continuously widening field of pragmatics as a means of providing further direction to assessment and treatment of aphasia in adults. Our initial effort in this regard was the development of Promoting Aphasics' Communicative Effectiveness (or PACE), which was introduced at the annual convention of the American Speech-Language-Hearing Association in 1978. This procedure is intended to structure treatment interaction according to components inherent to face-to-face conversation. This procedure has been attempted by clinicians on an international scale, and we have received many requests for complete information as to how to manage this procedure. However, since 1978 we have discovered that there is much more to pragmatics than conversational structure and, therefore, much more to pragmatic treatment than practicing conversation. Research delving into the relationships between language behavior and its contexts has taken off into a variety of areas that are still being discovered.

We are assuming that the reader already knows or has ready access to basic information about the nature of aphasia and standard rehabilitation procedures. This is not a comprehensive overview of aphasia rehabilitation. The audience for this book should be anyone interested in application of the study of language to clinical problems. However, we have two primary audiences in mind: (a) speech-language pathologists who are engaged in the assessment and treatment of aphasia in any clinical setting, and (b) students of speech-language pathology who may benefit from a supplemental text regarding a relatively new arena of clinical investigation. For the practicing clinician, we shall provide a scientifically supported rationale for the validity of pragmatic procedures that have been tried, as well as some new ideas for expanding rehabilitation into the realm of naturalistic language behavior. For the student, we have designed our discussion in part to reflect what we consider to be the logical steps in developing any type of clinical procedure.

Our suggestions for treatment are drawn from a model that delineates observable components of pragmatics and their relationship to language behavior. The book begins with an introduction to the pragmatic domain, in which relevant research with normal adults is cited. The next chapter presents investigations of aphasia as they pertain to the model of pragmatics. Such investigations provide insight into possible clinical procedures, which are initially discussed in Chapter 3 on assessment. In Chapter 4 treatment is presented first with a discussion of PACE, in which we elaborate on previous presentations of this procedure. Chapter 5 fills out remaining implications for treatment that are implied by the model of the pragmatic domain. Then Chapter 6 provides a few specific examples of PACE and other treatment suggestions in the form of case studies and some suggestions regarding group treatment of aphasic persons.

We received a great deal of assistance in completing this book, including the patient support of our colleagues at Memphis State University, the University of Massachusetts at Amherst, and Kent State University. We are grateful to Audrey Holland, Louise Ward, and Elizabeth Webster for the inspiration and understanding that they gave so freely as we developed the ideas in this book. Fortunately, we were able to repair early versions of the manuscript because of the insightful and thorough editing of Marilyn Newhoff. We want to thank the following students for their assistance in gathering references and compiling information: Tracy Griffith, Jennifer Barr, Nancy Meir, and Susan Gilbert. Finally, we wish to acknowledge the talented secretarial support of Shirley Rias and Susan Crites.

Chapter 1

Building a
Pragmatic Framework

Pragmatic aspects of communication (or simply "pragmatics") have received a great deal of recent attention in speech-language pathology. Its appearance has been similar to the wave of linguistics that swept over the profession during the 1960s and early 1970s. During that time, linguists and psycholinguists were informing clinicians about the nature of generative grammar and language "processing," and clinicians were attempting to create intervention protocols relevant to these concepts. Sometimes, the cart was put before the horse. That is, sensible applications preceded a thorough understanding of the normal processing of language; or they preceded basic research in the disorder; or programs were suggested before an application had been attempted. While putting the cart before the horse sounds like an unproductive thing to do, the apparently premature birth of a treatment program is not necessarily a mistake as long as the risks are recognized. Premature treatment programs can sometimes contribute to the development of a theoretical and factual framework, because the outcome of the application may modify or add to the foundation. Also, certain features of a treatment model may be so compelling and consistent with common sense that early application is inevitable. Such may be the case with pragmatics.

Pragmatics is *the study of the relationships between language behavior and the contexts in which it is used.* With respect to language users, these contexts may be characterized as external and internal. External contexts include situations in which language is used, and internal contexts include a person's emotional state and knowledge of the world. As a means of illustrating the communicative importance of contexts, let us consider the utterance "He did a Napoleon" (Clark and Gerrig, 1983). Various contextual parameters are necessary to understand what a speaker might mean by this utterance. One parameter is shared knowledge of the person being used in the verb phrase. The listener must know who Napoleon is. A second parameter might be a situation to which this utterance refers, such as making a portrait in a photographer's studio. In this case, familiarity with the famous painting of Napoleon would be brought to mind. Such utterances, in which speakers and listeners rely upon contextual variables, are common in everyday conversation.

In addition to examining contextual influences upon communicators' understanding of such phrases as "He did a Napoleon," researchers have begun to examine these influences in other types of communicative behavior, including indirect requests, metaphor, and idiom. Through these studies it has become apparent that a precise delineation of the domain of pragmatics is still in a process of evolution. This is evidenced by Rees' (1982) struggle to find a common thread underlying all the various definitions of pragmatics and her list of the various communicative phenomena that have been placed under "the umbrella heading of pragmatics" (e.g., speech acts, presupposition and inference, discourse operations, and social roles). When clinicians do their homework in order to learn about what is going on in the realm of pragmatics, they discover that current scholars and researchers are only beginning to understand the influences of contexts on language comprehension and production.

In this book, the main purposes are to review previous applications and to explore potential applications of pragmatics to rehabilitation of communicative functioning in adults with aphasia. These applications are discussed with respect to a comprehensive model that attempts to chart the domain of the pragmatic dimension of language behavior. Starting with a model as a frame of reference is necessary not only in order to understand clinical precedents but also in order to show what has been left out of consideration and, therefore, what is left to be done.

Ideally, the development of rehabilitation methods might procede as follows: (a) recognize a variable that has been determined to influence normal language processing or (b) determine that this variable can be a factor that influences aphasic performance or both; (c) create an idea for a treatment procedure that might capitalize on this factor; (d) actually carry out the task on a few clients, determining which clients are successful at it; (e) determine whether this success generalizes to genuine improvement in communicative abilities; and finally (f) present the procedure to the clinical world. We shall at least identify when we are leap-frogging from (a) to (c) to (f), recognizing the need, as Rosenbek (1979) so aptly put it, to trample through the intermediate steps acquiring wrinkled feet before we can be totally satisfied with what we have presented here. In effect, we hope that we raise more questions than we answer, and we hope to encourage many clinicians to begin applying and evaluating the effectiveness of a pragmatic model of treatment for persons with aphasia.

THE CONTEXTS OF LANGUAGE BEHAVIOR

We view context more broadly than it has been described in some previous investigations. For example, Winograd (1977) wrote that "pragmatic context" consists of the physical and social situation of participants in a conversation, but other contexts include knowledge and point of view of participants. We consider all of these contexts to rest beneath the umbrella of pragmatics. However, we do not wish to overextend the domain of pragmatics so that it necessarily includes the restricted, unnatural contexts of the traditional psycholinguistic laboratory (e.g., pictures to match with sentences, buttons to press). Rather, we wish to capture the spirit of pragmatics as reflecting contextual variables that are inherent to natural communicative interactions. In this sense, pragmatics absorbs contexts considered in sociolinguistics, such as participants, topic, and setting in a conversation (Ervin-Tripp, 1964; Freedle and Duran, 1979; Prutting, 1982; Robinson, 1972).

Our major contextual categories include linguistic, paralinguistic, and extralinguistic variables. These contexts not only determine the social appropriateness of language behavior, but also contribute to processing time and the meaning derived from an utterance. In our discussion of these three context categories, we treat them as separate entities for purposes of facilitating conceptualization. However, in a particular communicative interaction, it is difficult to attribute a listener's interpretation or a speaker's choice of utterance to only one of the many contextual variables that may be present. Hence, we ask our readers to keep in mind that these contexts interact in natural communicative situations and cannot be easily separated in reality.

Linguistic Context

Linguistic context is the verbal behavior that occurs before and after a given linguistic unit. It is studied at two levels: intrasentential context (relationships within a sentence) and intersentential context (relationships between sentences). Linguists refer to a series of sentences spoken in conversation or storytelling as *discourse*. Discourse is simply a "string of sentences." This definition is consistent with that of others who use the term to specify a level of linguistic inquiry (e.g., Winograd, 1977) rather than associating "discourse" with one type of communicative activity such as conversation (e.g., Roth and Spekman, 1984). When reading is studied, the linguistic level is identified as *text*. It is assumed that the structural properties of text and discourse are so similar that the study of text comprehension is used to generate conclusions about comprehension of oral discourse (Freedle, 1977, 1979; van Dijk and Kintsch, 1983).

Discourse is commonly divided into microstructural and macrostructural levels. According to Kintsch and van Dijk (1978), microstructure "is the local level of the discourse, that is, the structure of the individual propositions and their relations" (p. 365). Macrostructure, on the other hand, "is of a more global nature, characterizing the discourse as a whole" (p. 365). Both structural levels contribute to the *coherence* of a discourse. Because both levels involve the semantic structure of discourse, there is a hazy dividing line between formal linguistics and the domain of pragmatics.

Microstructure. Within a proposition or sentence, linguistic context can serve to disambiguate a lexical unit. For example, the effects of linguistic context on word comprehension have been examined frequently with respect to the comprehension of semantically ambiguous words (e.g., Foss and Jenkins, 1973; Swinney, 1979). Many words are semantically ambiguous by themselves or within a neutral context, such as the word "straw" in "The merchant put his straw beside the machine." Contexts that bias the meaning of an ambiguous word, as in "The farmer put his straw beside the machine," result in less time to process the ambiguous word than if the context were neutral (Foss and Jenkins, 1973).

At the intrasentential and intersentential levels, there are a number of devices used to maintain conversational coherence in general and referential coherence in particular. Referential coherence is critical for conversational coherence and refers to the overlap of argument among propositions. That is, two propositions are linked because they share one semantic element, as in the following: "A stroke is a disruption of blood supply to the brain. It frequently results in aphasia." With this example, we illustrated referential coherence at the intersentential level with the use of a pronoun that referred to a semantic element in the previous sentence (i.e., "stroke"). Referential coherence can also occur at the intrasentential level as in "The hunter shot himself." In this instance, a reflexive pronoun referred to a semantic element earlier in the sentence. More specifically, these examples illustrate the process of *coreference*, which is the dependence of a word or phrase upon previous linguistic context for its meaning. Pronouns provide a good example of coreference as they are inherently ambiguous and depend upon accurate and efficient identification of prior information for appropriate interpretation. They integrate discourse or text (e.g., Hirst and Brill, 1980); and a train of thought can be disrupted with pronoun selection, as in the following sequence:

(1a) The boys went to the zoo.
(1b) He fed the bears.

In another example of coreference, superordinate category terms (e.g., *vehicle*) might be used to refer to a specific subordinate category (e.g., *bus*) mentioned in a previous sentence. Articles, also, would help the listener know this, as in the following (Garrod and Sanford, 1977):

(2a) *A* bus came roaring around the corner.
(2b) *The* vehicle narrowly missed a pedestrian.

As indicated in 2a and 2b, articles assist in establishing links between sentences. A person uses "a" to refer to the first mention of an object or idea and uses "the" in subsequent references to the same object or idea. Therefore, "the" is a small cue that the referent is definitely one that was mentioned before, possibly in the previous sentence. For example, consider the use of articles in the following sequence:

(3a) A bus came roaring around the corner.
(3b) The bus hit a pedestrian.

The article in 3b indicates that it was the bus in 3a that hit the pedestrian. Misuse of articles can be illustrated by attempting to convey the same idea in the following manner:

(4a) A bus came roaring around the corner.
(4b) A bus hit a pedestrian.

In 4a and 4b, the speaker could have been referring to two different buses. Misuse of articles can be mildly startling and throw some confusion into a listener's or reader's attempt to remain on course as to what a speaker or writer is communicating (Irwin, Bock, and Stanovich, 1982).

A third type of bonding between two sentences is established when there is a causal relationship between them. Mandler and Johnson (1977) proposed that causally related statements are an especially powerful coherence device in narratives and that such statements would be easier to remember than those held together by other coherence devices or proximity. Black and Bern (1981) decided to test this proposal relative to temporally related statements, which are simply statements reflecting the sequence of events in a story. Subjects were asked to recall sentences from stories. These test sentences were preceded by another sentence that was in either a temporal relationship (5) or causal relationship (6) with the test sentence:

(5a) He lowered the flames and walked over to the refrigerator, seeing a bowl he had left on the table.
(5b) Suddenly it fell off the edge and broke.

(6a) He lowered the flames and walked over to the refrigerator, bumping
    a bowl he had left on the table.
(6b) Suddenly it fell off the edge and broke.

Black and Bern found that causally related events in a story were easier
to recall than temporally related events in a story.

The sentences in 6 show that only a one-word difference from 5a is
all that is needed to create a causal connection. Haberlandt and Bingham
(1978) examined the influence of word selection on intersentential
coherence. They demonstrated that by simply changing a verb in the middle
of a three-sentence triplet, a reader could be distracted from efficient
comprehension. Subjects were presented with coherent (7) and less coherent
(8) triplets, with coherency again being created by a causal relationship
(7b,c):

(7a) Brian punched George.
(7b) George called the doctor.
(7c) The doctor arrived.

(8a) Brian punched George.
(8b) George liked the doctor.
(8c) The doctor arrived.

Even though the third sentences (7c, 8c) were identical for each condition,
reading times for the these sentences were slower in the less coherent
condition (8), which did not contain a causal relationship between the
second and third sentences.

Macrostructure. Discourse or text consists of a global meaning (i.e.,
topic, theme) that contributes to intersentential coherence, thereby
facilitating comprehension. van Dijk (1977; Kintsch and van Dijk, 1978),
at the Univeristy of Amsterdam, has been a pioneer in the delineation of
the domains of linguistic macrostructure. He differentiated among
semantic, narrative, and pragmatic macrostructures. *Semantic*
macrostructure is a level of meaning consisting of constituent meanings
in a discourse. van Dijk defined a "macro-meaning" as "the unifying
property of the respective meanings of a sequence of propositions of a
discourse" (p. 7). "Macro-rules" are mapping rules applied to
microstructure to obtain macrostructure. "Generalization" is a macro-
rule that discovers the common meaning among propositions. While
semantic macrostructure lies in the domain of formal linguistics, our theme
in this book is more closely aligned with narrative and pragmatic
macrostructure.

According to van Dijk (1977), another kind of global structure may
be called "superstructures," one of which is a *narrative*. Narrative is one
of the most commonly analyzed superstructures (e.g., Thorndyke, 1977).
It is simply a story, "a discourse containing action sentences with specific
pragmatic conditions" (p. 16). Narrative macrostructures are conventional

in that the rules of storytelling belong to the general knowledge of language and culture shared by members of a community and, as such, are not by themselves linguistic. One of many examples of the organization of stories was studied by Kintsch (1977). Story constituents included such categories as "episode" sequences consisting of "an exposition, a complication, and a resolution." Other categories include a setting and a moral. Other superstructures include "procedural" discourse (Graesser, 1978) and the standard organization of a research article, which has been provided as an illustration of one kind of text grammar (Samuels and Eisenberg, 1981). Knowledge of superstructures has sometimes been called "narrative schemata," which are considered to be stored in long-term memory and employed in the processing of discourse or text in order to maximize the speed of comprehension (Kieras, 1978; Schank and Abelson, 1977).

Pragmatic macrostructure, according to van Dijk (1977), pertains to speech acts expressed by a discourse as well as the contributions of the situation and shared world knowledge to the global discourse meaning. For example, advice or an exhortation to buy a product may be the implied intention of a discourse that is not evident in its individual propositions but is inferred at the intersentential level. Also, participants and objects in the situation may contribute to global themes conveyed in coreference with personal and demonstrative pronouns. Shared world knowledge supplies implications drawn from macrostuctural topics or themes.

Paralinguistic Context

Paralinguistic context is "almost" language. It accompanies an utterance and its linguistic context. It is an inherent component of verbal productions, or what Prutting and Kirchner (1983) called the "trappings" surrounding a verbal production. General terminology includes suprasegmental features, intonation, and prosody. The history of research on this component of communication includes such classic works as Lieberman's (1967) acoustic and physiologic analyses of intonation and Goldman-Eisler's (1968) studies of hesitation pauses and their relationship to syntax and semantics. The term "prosody" has included intonation as one of its features. Barnes (1983) characterized prosody as rhythm, stress, and intonation that are the result of interaction among the measurable parameters of pitch, loudness, and duration. Other paralinguistic conventions include vocal quality, rate of speech, and juncture (i.e., brief pauses). Paralinguistic conventions serve a variety of purposes in communication. They are used to convey affective information and to formulate judgments about personality traits. They are also important to interpretation of utterance meanings and can be used to identify new information, to signal meaning of a word or phrase, and to identify the syntactic function of a statement.

Affect and Personality. The psychology of emotion (i.e., affect) has received a great deal of recent attention (e.g., Clark and Fiske, 1982; Collier, 1984). Paralinguistic parameters play a significant role in the communication of affective messages in English and probably many other languages (Laver and Trudgill, 1979; Williams and Stevens, 1972). For example, anger, in English, is frequently conveyed with a harsh vocal quality, elevated pitch and increased loudness; nervousness is frequently associated with an increased rate of speech. Investigation of affect and paralinguistic behavior has not been great in quanity and has often been hampered by the lack of objective analysis of paralinguistic parameters (Scherer, 1979). In general, the bulk of research in the area of paralinguistic communication has tended to focus less on the communication of affect and more on associations with and perceptions of specific personality traits.

Scherer (1979) conducted a detailed review of the various studies relating personality traits to paralinguistic behavior. A variety of research suggested a strong relationship between vocal quality (e.g., harsh, breathy, resonant) and such personality traits as emotional stability, introversion, and extroversion. Markel, Phillis, Vargas, and Howard (1972) found that rate (fast-slow) as well as intensity (loud-soft) were also associated with varying personality traits. In a slightly different vein, Brown, Strong, and Rencher (1974) and Smith, Brown, Strong, and Rencher (1975) found that perceptions of personality traits could be influenced by rate and pitch. Smith and coworkers demonstrated that ascription of the traits of "competence" and "benevolence" were influenced by rate of speech with an increased rate being associated with competence and a decreased rate being associated with benevolence. Brown and coworkers found that a decrease in pitch variance was associated with fewer ratings of competence and benevolence.

Utterance Meaning. Paralinguistic conventions are used in a variety of ways to aid or specify the meaning of an utterance. One application involves focusing a listener upon new information in a sentence or a discourse. For example, let us consider the following sentences in which stress is used to identify the new information.

(9a) Harrison ate the *squid*.
(9b) *Harrison* ate the squid.

With 9a, the speaker has assumed that the listener already knows that Harrison ate something but does not know what he ate. Stress is used to highlight the new information. In 9b, in which stress is also used to highlight the new information, the speaker has assumed that the listener already knows that someone ate the squid but not who. The two examples illustrate the way in which a paralinguistic variable (i.e., stress) is manipulated to convey different meaning in otherwise identical sentences.

Paralinguistic conventions may also be used to signal semantic interpretations or to facilitate syntactic analysis of a word or phrase. For example, a statement may be turned into a question with a rising pitch at the end. In the sentence "They are fighting dogs," stress and juncture determine whether "fighting" is to be interpreted as a modifier or a verb. These prosodic features, therefore, provide surface structural cues to the deep structure of an utterance. A common example of the need for prosodic cues to deep structure comes from contemplating three possible meanings of "Time flies like an arrow" (Sowa, 1983):

> (10a) Time (noun) flies (verb) like an arrow.
> (10b) Time flies (noun phrase) like an arrow.
> (10c) Time (verb) flies (noun) like an arrow.

While some of these meanings are unusual, they are possible given a creative linguistic context generated from a peculiar imagination. This example refers to time that flies (10a), time flies that are fond of something (10b), and recording the speed of flies (10c).

As another example of semantic-syntactic prosody, syllabic stress may be necessary to identify whether "convict" is a noun or a verb. Stress and juncture differentiate "sorehead" from "sore head." Juncture helps a listener to determine whether someone is saying "Watch it swing" or "Watch its wing." Of course, if we were to imagine the actual use of these words and sentences, our imagination would include linguistic or situational contexts or both that would facilitate interpretation. Perhaps, the only time such utterances would appear in isolation, thereby demanding help from paralinguistic conventions, would be in a study or clinical assessment of prosodic abilities.

Extralinguistic Context

Extralinguistic context is an elusive and powerful determiner of communicative behavior. It is elusive in the sense that contextual components and their interactions with each other are difficult to identify. Identification is difficult, partly because the important components frequently vary from culture to culture (Brown and Fraser, 1979). For example, some cultures regard hugging and kissing as an appropriate form of greeting, but other cultures might regard such behavior as too demonstrative. This elusiveness is compounded because extralinguistic context is multifaceted. It includes gestures, knowledge of a topic, and the situation in which a communicative interchange occurs. Extralinguistic context can be regarded as powerful because it usually governs *what* message is communicated, *how* a message is communicated, and *when* a message is communicated. Several investigators have described parameters of extralinguistic context (e.g., Brown and Fraser, 1979; Giles, Scherer, and Taylor, 1979; Prutting and Kirchner, 1983). These parameters are classified with respect to the purpose, the setting, and the participants associated with a communicative exchange. We have summarized these extralinguistic parameters in Table 1-1. We shall refer to this list in subsequent chapters, since it guides the planning of treatment that incorporates extralinguistic variables.

Purposes. Purposes can be characterized with respect to general types of activities that may serve as a focal point for interpersonal communication (Brown and Fraser, 1979). Examples of general activity types include sports events, teaching, shopping, chatting with a friend, and conducting a meeting. Each of these activities may entail characteristic goals such as motivating a listener to improve an effort, instructing someone as to how to do something, obtaining something from someone else, ventilating feelings, pleasing another person, and so on.

The style and content of an utterance may vary as a function of the different goals of different activities. A form that is appropriate in one situation may not be appropriate in another. For example, imagine a frustrated football coach saying the following to an assistant during a game: "It would appear that the official made an error in penalizing our number 38 for clipping." While we do not need to put into print the more likely form of this message for the coach's purpose in this situation, we could imagine that this statement would have more likely been made during a class in which students were learning the rules of football. However, the interactive elusiveness of context comes into play with this contrived example, because, given a twist of prosody, this statement might be heard in the heat of battle as an extreme sarcasm. Besides linguistic form, other aspects of communication may be tied to purpose of an interaction, such as turn-taking conventions in a conversation. If a conversation is for conducting business in a formal meeting, there may not be as many interruptions of turns as there would be in a chat between friends.

Discourse structure may also be influenced by the purpose of a communicative interaction. Let us consider a conversation that involves everything that participants know about weasels. A speaker's purpose might be to instruct a listener on the care and feeding of a weasel. This instruction would have the characteristic structure of procedural discourse, consisting of a sequence of essential and optional steps (Ulatowska, Doyel, Stern, Haynes, and North, 1983). Another purpose might simply be to inform a listener about a recent experience with a weasel, and such a description would possess the structure of narrative discourse.

Table 1-1. Extralinguistic Parameters

Purpose

    Activity type: shopping, meeting, chatting
    Subject matter: price of pork, tennis etiquette, aphasia

Setting

    Place: home, church, work, store, clinic
    Physical surroundings: rain, hills, an elevator
    Bystanders
    Time: early morning, late afternoon
    General: formal, informal

Participants

    Conceptual knowledge (shared)
        Facts about the world
        Social mores
    Emotional state
    Roles
        Group identification: religion, race, sex, subculture
        Familiarity/kinship/authority: spouse, minister, clinician
    Physical orientation: face-to-face, side-by-side
    Movements: postural, differential (e.g., gestures)

Setting. The setting of a communicative interaction includes physical and temporal parameters. These parameters include the place (e.g., grocery store), surroundings (e.g., steep hill, snow), time of day (e.g., morning, afternoon), and the presence or absence of persons who are not participating in the conversation. A given setting may direct style of conversation and lexical selection. For example, people may talk a certain way because they are in a church, in another person's home, or are walking across sacred ground. Knowledge of the rules for talking in different situations forms part of what is called "social competence" (Prutting, 1982). People conform to such rules as "Don't talk loud in church" or "I don't talk much early in the morning." People may use one set of vocabulary at work in the mill and another set of vocabulary with the family at the dinner table.

A broad dimension that characterizes variations of setting is formality. Style and content of verbalizations vary between formal and informal settings. Places may be defined as being typically formal or informal, for example, the chief executive's suite or the gymnasium's locker room, respectively. However, formality may be determined by the personal tastes and styles of persons using a place. For example, a business office may be formal or informal; a person's home may be formal or informal; a speech-language clinic may have a formal or informal atmosphere. Clinicians may or may not wear white jackets because of the atmosphere they wish to create. Because environments outside of the clinic vary in formality, a clinic that fosters only one style does not reflect what the client must deal with elsewhere.

Participants. Participants bring a variety of dimensions to a communicative interaction that are independent of utterances spoken in the interaction. These contexts are internal and external relative to a participant in a conversation and they include (a) conceptual knowledge possessed by each participant, (b) the emotional state of each participant, (c) the role of each participant, (d) physical orientation of participants to each other, and (e) movements produced by each participant. Discussion of emotional state is presented in Chapter 2.

The contribution of knowledge can be depicted by the simple notion that comprehension is aided when a listener knows something about what a speaker is talking about. *Prior knowledge* of phonological theory is helpful when listening to someone talk about stridency. Howard Cosell is easier to understand when a listener knows something about boxing. The word "grout" is likely to be understood by someone with a knowledge of building construction, and this word is most likely to be produced by someone who knows something about building construction. *Attitudes* toward a topic and a speaker may also influence attention, comprehension, and memory when listening to a speech or a speaker in a conversation. When the topic is boxing, a like or dislike for this subject (and a like or dislike for Howard Cosell) determines attention and recall. In a study involving paragraphs about the Soviet Union, ability to recall paragraphs was influenced favorably by prior knowledge and a positive attitude toward the topic (Tyler and Voss, 1982). The fact that prior knowledge is used during cognitive processing was indicated in a study showing that it takes up "space" in working memory (Britton and Tesser, 1982).

In a conversation, prior knowledge is included within a dimension designated as *shared knowledge*. When both participants know something about building construction, "grout" may be produced and understood by either participant. Success of communication in a conversation is determined partly by the degree to which participants share knowledge of the topic. The power of this variable can be imagined by considering an aphasic individual talking with a clinician, spouse, or stranger about (a) a treatment plan, (b) a family vacation, or (c) the major news of the day. All one has to do is imagine different combinations of participants and topics. Communication may be more successful between client and clinician about a treatment plan than between the same participants about a family vacation. Communication may be more successful between client and spouse about a family vacation than between the same participants about a treatment plan. People tend to talk with strangers about news events, because there is a greater likelihood of shared knowledge with such topics. These examples are intended to indicate that the success of communication between a clinician and a client is not solely dependent upon the client's linguistic abilities but may also rely, to a large degree, on shared knowledge.

The examples in the previous paragraph included *role* variation in the imagined conversational participants. Roles can be identified in two ways. One involves characteristics that distinguish individuals from each other, and another involves variations of role that can be assumed by a single individual. The former is related to a person's identification with a particular group that may be socially or culturally based (e.g., Hippies of the 1960s, Valley girls of the 1980s) or occupationally based (e.g., physician, sportscaster, professor). A speaker may adopt a linguistic or pragmatic style that is characteristic of the group (Rosch, 1977). A listener may interpret an utterance differently depending on whether it is spoken by a liberal politician or a conservative minister.

The second identification of role pertains to the social relationship between participants in a conversation. Communicative variations have been observed as a function of familiarity, kinship, and perceived authority (Brown and Fraser, 1979). Linguistic and pragmatic style may vary, depending on whether the participants are adult-child, mother-daughter, husband-wife, employer-employee, and so on (e.g., Freedle, Naus, and Schwartz, 1977). Freedle and Duran (1979) explained how these sociolinguistic variables might affect code selection, paralinguistic devices, the sequencing of comments in a dialogue, and choice of message form. Group characteristics and social role contribute to rules of social competence such as "Never talk to your mother that way."

Physical orientation refers to whether participants might be facing each other, standing side-by-side, or back-to-back. It also refers to distance between participants. To a certain degree physical orientation is determined by the general activity type. For example, in a lecture there is usually a predetermined distance between speaker and listeners, and the speaker is facing the listeners. At a formal dinner many participants will typically be seated side by side. At parties people tend to cluster in small groups in which participants are facing each other. In other situations, distance between communicators varies as a funtion of familiarity and comfort with the situation. There are clear linguistic correlates of distance between communicators, and these are typically related to loudness (Brown and Fraser, 1979). Linguistic correlates of physical orientation have also been examined. Moscovici and Plon (cited in Brown and Fraser, 1979) found that speech in side-to-side and back-to-back interactions tended to be more nominal than when participants were facing each other.

Movement can be postural or differentiated. Postural movements include forward and backward leans. Differentiated movements include limb gestures, facial expression, and gaze direction. These movements may accompany verbal behavior as a means of regulating elements of conversation such as turn-taking (Rosenfeld, 1978). Other types of differentiated movement are communicative, as supplements or substitutes for verbal behavior. In normal conversation, they are generally supplemental and, therefore, provide a portion of the context for linguistic behavior. Gestures may function as symbols or signals, and recognition of their variety is important for analyzing their use (see Chapter 3). Symbolic gestures refer to objects and actions, and they may be arbitrary representations or direct representations (e.g., pantomime). Signals are generally unintentional displays of emotion or responses to stimuli (e.g., scratching an itch). Intentionality can be definitive, because the "scratching an itch" movement may be used as a symbol to convey heavy thinking or a degree of confusion. Formal symbolic gesture systems may be considered to be languages that are subjected to the same influences of context as verbal language.

Summary of Contexts

Various manifestations of linguistic, paralinguistic, and extralinguistic contexts have been reviewed. Linguistic context maintains the coherence of discourse at microstructural and macrostructural levels. At the microstructural level, coherence is achieved with articles and clear pronoun coreference. At the macrostructural level, the topic of a discourse can hold several sentences together. Paralinguistic context conveys a speaker's mood or emotional state, and it serves as cues to meaning and sentence form. Extralinguistic context is most commonly associated with "pragmatics"; it includes the situation, conversational participants' status and roles, their world knowledge, and their movements. These contexts blend with each other in natural communicative situations, as when success of communication depends upon shared knowledge and the situation (e.g., comprehending "He did a Napoleon"). Classifying these naturally merging components should assist researchers and clinicians in investigating, evaluating, and managing identifiable variables—even those that contribute to "natural" events.

CONTEXT IN ACTION

The three major contexts have been presented as somewhat static entities that may have an effect on linguistic processing. Now we turn our attention to the dynamics of conversation, showing how contexts influence the exchange of messages by participants in communicative interaction. After presenting essential elements of conversation, we shall address two special interactions between context and language, namely, distinguishing between given and new information and conveying and comprehending intended meaning. Each of the three general classes of context play a role in affecting these two interactions.

Conversation

The interaction structure of conversation differs from traditional laboratory (and clinical) interactions between subject and experimenter (or between subject and machine). Formal investigation of conversation usually involves the study of two participants, a unit commonly referred to as the conversational *dyad*. Participants follow certain rules that manage who speaks and who listens and that prohibit participants from talking at the same time. Also, formulation of messages is based on a central assumption shared by participants in a conversation.

The Cooperative Principle. Conversation is normally a cooperative endeavor in which each participant recognizes a common purpose or shares the direction of this endeavor. The assumption of cooperation comprises "a type of social contract" inherent to conversation (Clark and Haviland, 1977). Grice's (1975) delineation of the cooperative principle has become a basis for explaining interactions between language and context that are discussed in the next two sections (i.e., distinguishing given and new information and conveying nonliteral meanings). According to Grice, cooperation is achieved by following four *maxims*: (a) make your contribution no more or less informative than is required for the purpose of the exchange, (b) try to be truthful, conveying what you believe or have adequate evidence for, (c) be relevant to the topic, and (d) be easy to understand by being orderly and by avoiding ambiguity and obscurity.

The results of language production and comprehension are determined, in part, by following the four maxims. A speaker constructs an utterance based on *presuppositions* about what the listener already knows. The speaker "takes the point of view" of the listener. In requesting "Please, do a Napoleon for the camera," a photographer assumes that the subject is familiar with a portrait of Napoleon (Clark and Gerrig, 1983). If the photographer does not make this presupposition and uses this directive anyway, he or she risks a failure in communication by violating the obscurity maxim. In another instance, a speaker may appear to be violating the truth maxim by remarking that "It sure is hot in here" when actually it is quite cold. However, assuming that the social contract of cooperation is in effect, a listener would assume that the speaker is trying to be truthful. Usually such a violation is only apparent. According to Grice (1975), the listener would draw a *conversational implicature* and, in doing so, would simply figure out what the speaker meant. The speaker may be using irony in order to convey a feeling as to how cold it seems to be. There are three essential elements in this communication: one is the utterance; another is the situational context; and the third is the social contract of cooperation, all of which contribute to the meaning that is conveyed.

Conversational Moves. An essential characteristic of conversation is *turn-taking* between participants in which each person alternates in roles of sender and receiver of information. This alternation has been called "the reciprocity rule" (Jaffe, 1978) or "role-complementarity" (Rosenfeld, 1978). While persons' talking at the same time is somewhat anarchistic, Jaffe argued, also, that the nervous system is not built to handle simultaneous speaking and listening by an individual.

We shall borrow liberally from the terminology of Weiner and Goodenough (1977) in our description of conversational behavior. They described the conversation "game" as being a series of "moves" taken according to certain rules. Characteristics of conversation can be divided into two broad categories: (a) "housekeeping moves" that are somewhat independent of the conveyance of messages and (b) "substantive moves" that contribute directly to the transmission of content from one participant to another. While Weiner and Goodenough focused on the utterance as the minimal unit for a move, conversational moves can also be nonverbal or gestural.

Housekeeping moves are used to manage turn-taking in a conversational interaction. They have also been called "regulators" (Harrison, 1974; Rosenfeld, 1978). Gestural housekeeping behavior has been called "gesticulation" and has been described as serving conversational control functions (Rosenfeld, 1978). Gestural behavior is particularly important in the control of turning-taking, by establishing initiation of a speaker turn, maintenance of the speaker role, and switching roles from listener to speaker or vice versa. Eye gaze (i.e., shifting away from the listener) and hand movements are used by a participant to initiate and maintain a speaking turn. Boundaries of speaker and listener turns serve to identify units of observation in the investigation of conversation. Pioneering "linguistic" description of turn-taking was developed by Sacks, Schegloff, and Jefferson (1974) with early studies of turn-taking conducted by Duncan (1972; Duncan and Niederehe, 1974).

Weiner and Goodenough (1977) showed that turn-taking procedures vary according to the relative status of participants in a conversational dyad. In defining their parameters, these investigators developed some unique terminology in relating turn-taking to topic continuation and shifting. They described the "passing move" as a housekeeping device designed to shift the topic. The passing move is "a turn or part of a turn in which the utterer relinquishes his option to make a substantive contribution to the topic talk of the conversation at that moment. . ." (p. 217). The other participant may continue the topic, shift the topic, or make another passing move creating the "passing move pair." Rules become more precise with two types of passing moves: (a) the "OK pass" by which a listener gives up a speaking turn and allows the speaker to continue, and (b) the "repetition pass" in which one participant simply repeats or paraphrases the other participant's discourse. A passing move that occupies an entire turn was called a "passing turn"; one that occupies part of a turn was called a "framing move," and so on.

Weiner and Goodenough (1977) studied interactions between participants with unequal status, such as doctor-patient and teacher-student dyads. They found that unilateral framing moves occur frequently in the speech of high-status participants, do not occur often in peer interactions, and are rarely used by low-status participants. That is, high-status speakers appear to take more control than low-status participants in signaling topic shifts. The passing move pair, when the other participant passes after the speaker has passed, occurs in peer interactions as an explicitly mutual designation of a topic shift. This study offers one example of how a component of extralinguistic context influences extralinguistic communicative behavior, as well as offering a means of identifying behaviors to facilitate assessment of conversation.

We shall consider *substantive moves* to be those that contribute to the conveyance of messages. A conversation begins with one participant taking a speaking turn and attempting to convey a message with the best form that comes to mind at the time (e.g., "How about them Cubbies!"). At the same time, the other participant assumes the role of listener, attempting to comprehend the intended meaning of the speaker (e.g., *Hmm. I wonder what he's really after*). Sometimes the listener does not understand the speaker's message, an occurrence that is called a communicative "breakdown." The listener responds with a move called a *contingent query* (e.g., "What? Who are the Cubbies?") (Garvey, 1979). The source of the breakdown could be the speaker, who may make a faulty presupposition about the listener's knowledge; or it could be the listener who may not be paying attention. The speaker may reform the message in response to the query (e.g., "What do you think about Chicago's baseball team?"), until the message is conveyed to the listener (e.g., "Oh. I don't pay much attention to baseball").

Communication obstacles are common when one participant has a language disorder, such as aphasia. An impaired speaker often has difficulty getting his or her idea across on the first attempt, what Lubinski called a "hint" that starts a *hint-and-guess* conversational cycle (Lubinski, Duchan, and Weitzner-Lin, 1980). Several outcomes are possible in these sequences: *resolution*, in which the speaker confirms that the listener's guess was the speaker's intended meaning; *breakdown*, in which the listener makes an incorrect guess that is indicated by the speaker's reply; *revision*, in which the speaker modifies his or her original attempt after acknowledging that a breakdown had occurred; and *repair*, in which the speaker improves his or her utterance after the listener has provided a correct interpretation.

Conveying Given and New Information

The cooperative principle specifies that comprehenders and speakers adhere to certain conventions in a conversation. These conventions include the "maxims" cited in the previous section. While a speaker is "being cooperative" by following these maxims, a listener comprehends based on his or her assumption that the speaker is being cooperative. The listener assumes, for example, that the speaker is being informative. This assumption is a part of the social contract for conversation that Clark and Haviland (1977) called the *given-new contract* which, they concluded, plays a central role in the comprehension of sentences (and in the production of sentences, as well). That is, intended meaning is conveyed because of the listener's assumption that the speaker is conveying new information. The speaker, in fact, has certain syntactic conventions available that help the listener to identify new information. Even if the speaker does not appear to be conveying new information by using appropriate syntactic rules, the listener assumes that the speaker is being cooperative and still looks for new information by conversational implicature.

A speaker constructs sentences so that they are "congruent with his knowledge of the listener's mental world" (Clark and Haviland, 1977, p. 4). A speaker distinguishes between *given* information, namely, information that is known to a listener, and *new* information, namely, information that is novel to a listener. Given information is derived from a speaker's presupposition about what a listener already knows. Clark and Haviland stated that at the heart of the given-new contract is the "maxim of antecedence," which specifies that clues in an utterance to given information should be unambiguous. If they are ambiguous, a listener will use certain procedures to find given information in his or her world knowledge. Haviland and Clark (1974) suggested that sentence comprehension involves relating new information to given information.

They found that comprehension is best facilitated when given information is presented directly in a preceding sentence than when it must be inferred.

Various linguistic and paralinguistic conventions are used to distinguish between given and new information (MacWhinney and Bates, 1978). *Contrastive stress* is used on any element of a sentence to signify new information, as in the following:

(11) Romeo *kissed* Juliet.

This utterance implies that the listener already knows that Romeo did something to Juliet and is being informed that Romeo kissed her. Special syntactic constructions may be used when the listener knows that someone kissed Juliet but does not know who kissed her, as in the *cleft construction* of 12:

(12) It was Romeo who kissed Juliet.
(13) It was Romeo who kissed her.

When information is already given, *ellipsis* is used whereby the given information is omitted, for example, in answering "Who kissed Juliet?" (e.g., "Romeo"). *Pronominalization* signifies given information (e.g., 13). Earlier in this chapter, we showed how pronouns maintain coherence among a series of sentences (e.g., "Juliet was kissed last night in her boudoir. It was Romeo who kissed her"). Pronoun reference to given information is also a device of referential coherence. While reading a paragraph, processing of a pronoun such as "her" is faster when it is close to the antecedent than when it is separated from the antecedent by a couple of sentences (Ehrlich and Rayner, 1983).

In maintaining coherence, articles also distinguish between given and new information, as in 14:

(14a) An admirer was hanging around beneath Juliet's balcony.
(14b) She dropped a potted plant on the brash young man's head.
(14c) She dropped a potted plant on a brash young man's head.

In 14a, the indefinite article "an" signifies new information. The definite article "the" in 14b informs a listener that the victim is already known and probably is the loitering admirer. A listener could not be certain of this if 14c were heard instead of 14b, because a listener expects "a" to signal new information; 14c is suggestive of the possibility that the admirer and the young man are two different people. Appropriate use of "a" to signify new information and "the" to signify given information are significantly faster to process than their inappropriate use to signify given and new information, respectively (Irwin et al., 1982).

Investigators have been interested for some time in observing the effect of the given-new contract on verbal behavior. Making such observations involves setting up a condition in which a speaker must convey new information to a listener and also is continually making assumptions about what the listener already knows. If these assumptions change, then new information should be modified accordingly. Investigators arrange what we shall call a *new information condition*, in which a listener is shielded from view of objects or pictures that a speaker has been asked to describe to the listener. One of the earliest attempts to arrange a new information condition was in studies of children in which a screen prohibited visual contact between a speaker and listener as a speaker instructed a listener to stack different blocks (e.g., Glucksberg and Krauss, 1967). In a study that shielded adult listeners from speakers, Krauss and Weinheimer (1964) found that, as listeners were told more and more about an abstract geometric figure, the adult speakers decreased the number of descriptive labels used to enable listeners to identify what was being described. A speaker makes such adjustments because of his or her presuppositions about what the listener already knows from previous descriptions.

The Speaker's Meaning

Quite often, if not typically, in conversation a speaker does not literally mean what is said. To be polite, a speaker may make a request indirectly, as in "Can you open the door?" or "It's been a long time since I have been to a movie." Also, comparisons are frequently made that are not literally true (e.g., "This test is a bear"; "The world is a stage"; "Bubba is a Neanderthal"). Certain falsehoods become quite common (e.g., "He kicked the bucket"; "She buried the hatchet"; "They are shooting the bull"). Statements that can be true may become literally false as when, in an air-conditioned room filled with arguing Republicans and Democrats, someone observes "It sure is getting hot in here." This message appears to be truthful. There can be a "heated debate," "lonely heart," or "cheerful trumpet." The study of such utterances falls within the province of pragmatics, because in many instances a listener must rely on internal and external contexts in order to comprehend a speaker's meaning. Meaning may not be found in a mental dictionary of word-referent relationships. A listener must figure out what a speaker is saying. Natural communication is filled with idiom, metaphor, and irony; therefore, a complete theory of language comprehension and production should account for these forms.

Traditional linguistics and psycholinguistics have consisted of the study of literal meaning and syntactic creativity. Literal meaning involves the semantic interpretation of a sentence by itself, without any special relationship to its use by different speakers in different situations. Searle

(1969) referred to this content as the "proposition." Syntactic creativity has been seen as the potential for production of an infinite number of different sentences because of the generative power of a few rules of syntax. However, language users are capable of infinite semantic creativity, as well, by utilizing shared knowledge and the situation in relation to sentences, in order to convey ideas and impressions that are not contained literally in a sentence (Paivio, 1979).

Speech act theory was developed to distinguish between the literal content of a proposition and its intended or conveyed meaning (Searle, 1969). Conveyed meaning was called the "illocutionary force" of an utterance. Speech acts were considered to be basic units of communication. These units include asserting, requesting, advising, questioning, and greeting. The form of a proposition may differ from the speech act conveyed with that proposition, as when a request is conveyed with a question form. More recently, Searle (1979) and others (e.g., Morgan, 1979) have distinguished between *sentence meaning* and *speaker meaning,* also "utterance meaning," when discussing the distinction between literal and nonliteral interpretation, respectively. The new terminology reflects the ideas that interpretation involves more than the identification of a speech act (e.g., in metaphor) and that utterance meaning involves examination of what a speaker does with a sentence. There is a genuine relationship between symbols and users in which intended meaning of word, phrase, or sentence cannot be found in a dictionary but is a creation in the mind of a speaker.

Indirect Requests. A speaker's intent, in the form of a speech act, may differ from the literal form and interpretation of an utterance. The indirect request has been a common vehicle for studying the role of this difference in language behavior. A mother's request to straighten up a room may be conveyed with a statement form (e.g., "I can't stand this mess in here") or with an interrogative form (e.g., "Can you clean up your room?") instead of the more direct imperative form (e.g., "For the last time, straighten up this mess!"). Response to indirect requests may involve conversational implicature, because the cooperation maxim of relevance appears to be violated when someone is apparently asking about ability to straighten up a room. The assumption of cooperation compels a listener to consider context in order to determine what a speaker really means.

Clark and Lucy (1975) proposed a model for comprehension of indirect speech acts that involves three processing stages: first, a listener makes a literal interpretation of an utterance; second, determines whether the utterance is consistent with its context; and, third, if the utterance is inconsistent with context, infers a nonliteral interpretation based on the comparison with context. However, Gibbs (1981, 1982) argued that there are conventional forms of indirect request that, in conventional contexts, require fewer processing stages than the number suggested in the three-stage model. "Can you . . ." is a conventional indirect request form, while "Is it possible for you to clean up your room?" is unconventional. Gibbs found that people take less time to comprehend conventional indirect requests than unconventional indirect requests. Certain forms of indirect request may be understood as automatically as literal statements or direct requests, without an intervening stage involving a literal interpretation.

Metaphor. Metaphor has also become a means of studying language-context interactions through differences between sentence meaning and speaker meaning. It is often easy to recognize but difficult to define (Ortony, Reynolds, and Arter, 1978). Metaphor might be defined as "a figure of speech" that suggests a likeness by speaking of something as if it were something else. To say that "Bubba is a Neanderthal" is to suggest that Bubba is like a Neanderthal or that he shares certain attributes of Neanderthals. In following the cooperative principle, a speaker of this utterance would assume that a listener is being cooperative and knows something about Neanderthals. The listener, assuming that the speaker is being truthful, searches his or her knowledge of the paleolithic period of evolution in order to comprehend. Therefore, it is understood through implicature that the speaker is making a comparison and is conveying a truth about Bubba in a way that connotes more than just "Bubba is rather primitive." Metaphor is a synergy between language and context, creating a new idea through the integration of established ideas.

A few attempts have been made to analyze the components of a metaphor. Searle (1979) explained that a linguistic theory of metaphor should state the principles by which sentence meaning is related to nonliteral or speaker meaning. Authors have utilized a breakdown by Richards (1936), who stated that a metaphor consists of a *topic* (subject term, e.g., "Bubba"), a *vehicle* (term being used metaphorically, e.g., "Neanderthal"), and a *ground* (the relationship between topic and vehicle, e.g., primitiveness). The relationship between topic and vehicle may possess a *tension* due to their logical incompatibility. Searle (1979) provided a similar description with S is P as the sentence and S is R as the metaphorical or speaker's meaning. In these linguistic descriptions, "S" is the topic (subject term), "P" is the vehicle, and "R" is the meaning of the vehicle that the speaker is relating to the topic. Just to provide an idea of Searle's principles for relating sentence and speaker meaning, we shall mention two of them:

(a)   "Things which are P are by definition R. Usually, if the metaphor
       works, R will be one of the salient defining characteristics of P ";
(b) "Things which are P are often said or believed to be R, even though
       both speaker and hearer may know that R is false of P." (p. 116)

There are different types of metaphor, and these differences become
important in understanding how metaphor might be processed. Each of
the following statements can be a metaphor:

(15a) This omelet is a brick.
(15b) She buried the hatchet.
(16a) It is cold in here.
(16b) Regardless of the danger, the troops marched on.

The common feature of the statements in 15 is that both can be recognized
as being metaphors without knowledge of a special context. The difference
between these statements is that 15a is not possible in the real world and
15b is possible, but not plausible. Also, 15b is used so commonly that
it has become an idiom and, therefore, is immediately understood with
respect to its speaker or nonliteral meaning. The feature shared by the
statements in 16 is that both are not obviously metaphors. Their literal
meaings are possible and plausible. These statements may become
metaphors because of the way in which they are used by a speaker in order
to convey something else. As a description of two persons seated at each
end of a sofa and not speaking to each other, 16a becomes a metaphor.
In a study of the influence of context on language comprehension, Ortony,
Schallert, Reynolds, and Antos (1978) placed statements such as 16b after
written contexts such as a description of a babysitter trying unsuccessfully
to control an unruly group of children. With such a context, 16b becomes
a metaphor with its nonliteral meaning.

Some terminology for the distinctions among metaphors has been
introduced in the literature on language behavior. Metaphors such as 15b
are called *dead* or *stored* metaphors, and sometimes are referred to as
"idioms." Idioms may vary in their degree of "frozenness" depending
on how well their nonliteral meaning holds up when they are transformed,
as from active to passive form (Swinney and Cutler, 1979). The many
examples of dead metaphor or idiom include "He kicked the bucket,"
"They let off some steam," "She faced the music," and "He hit the
ceiling." While varying in their real-world plausibility, nonliteral
interpretation of such utterances appears to be understood more quickly
than literal interpretation (Ortony, Schallert, Reynolds, and Antos, 1978).
Sometimes nonliteral interpretation is automatic, rendering a three-stage
model of comprehension, such as Clark and Lucy's for indirect requests,
irrelevant for some metaphors in some situations (Gildea and Glucksberg,

1983; Glucksberg, Gildea, and Bookin, 1982). Statements such as 15a, on the other hand, appear to be creative expressions that must be "figured out" on the spot by a listener. These are called *fresh* metaphors (Morgan, 1979; Ortony, Reynolds, and Arter, 1978), and a three-stage model of nonliteral comprehension may be relevant for them.

A third type of metaphor, represented by 16a and 16b, is recognized for its nonliteral interpretation only within a certain context, when a speaker has decided to use an ordinary statement metaphorically. We refer to these as *context-dependent* metaphors. In any case, the meanings of metaphors cannot be described with a traditional semantic theory. These meanings are aroused, especially with fresh and context-dependent metaphor, depending on how a speaker uses a sentence with respect to shared knowledge of the world and a particular situational context.

SUMMARY AND CONCLUSION

In our introductory chapter, we have put together a variety of definitions and investigations that have dealt with the interaction between language behavior and context, thereby, presenting the first step of our idealized strategy for developing treatment methods. In doing so, we have attempted to map out the domain of pragmatics as a study of language—a framework that should guide investigators in studying the pragmatic abilities of aphasic persons, as well as in developing pragmatic approaches to clinical assessment and treatment. We identified three types of context as being linguistic, paralinguistic, and extralinguistic. We described parameters of the most common behavioral structure in which these contexts are used, namely, the conversational dyad. The principal characteristic of this communicative interaction is turn-taking between participants. The social contract of cooperation between participants in a conversation leads to making distinctions between given and new information and contributes to the effective use of indirect requests, metaphor, and other linguistic behaviors in which speaker meaning differs from sentence meaning. The relationships between language behavior and language users indeed are central to understanding how language works as a mode of communication in natural environments.

Chapter 2

Communicative Behavior in Aphasic Adults

Chapter 1 was introduced with an idealized sequence of steps for the development of rehabilitation methods. While the first chapter dealt with the first step (i.e., determining effects of context on normal language behavior), the second chapter includes a consideration of the second step, namely, determining effects of context on aphasic language behavior. Furthermore, the second chapter focuses on the effect of focal damage in the left cerebral hemisphere on pragmatic aspects of communicative behavior.

The present chapter has a more direct bearing on the development of assessment and treatment strategies that are sensitive to language-context interactions. While studies of normal adults are indicative of how a particular pragmatic function might be tested and exercised, studies of aphasic persons are indicative of the procedures that are likely to elicit successful communicative behaviors from different clients. Often the methods of cognitive psychology are too difficult for brain-injured persons, and these methods must be "scaled down" so that the target behavior can be observed clearly and different levels of success can be measured.

Just as the normal language processor operates in concert with its contexts, the damaged language processor must attempt to interact with internal and external contexts in order to achieve communication. Aphasia has been viewed as being a primary disruption of language behavior, leaving internal and external contexts relatively intact (e.g., Davis, 1983). In a sense, contexts outside of the patient remain as they were before impairment had occurred, except for disruptions to interpersonal interaction and lives of family members. Focal damage may interact more directly with internal contexts, such as emotions and conceptual knowledge. Components of cognition are interconnected, as are regions of the brain. A lesion may corrupt operation of nearby regions. The primary cognitive deficit may lie at a depth that is common to the processing of nonverbal and verbal input. Therefore, it is possible that recognition and production of contexts, as well as of language-context interactions, are affected by injury to the language regions of the brain.

On the other hand, untarnished regions of the brain are responsible for certain strengths remaining in an aphasic person's communicative ability. These strengths are found in remaining levels of linguistic functions, compensatory linguistic behaviors, and active and passive uses of contexts. Research on pragmatics and aphasia has pointed out a few deficits that had not been considered before and has pointed out some strengths in patients' communicative ability that had not been emphasized before. With respect to the domain of pragmatics, large gaps in our knowledge of language-context relationships exist in the study of communicative function in aphasia. We intend to point out these gaps, in order to encourage expansion of current pragmatically oriented investigations.

LINGUISTIC CONTEXT: DISCOURSE AND TEXT

Questions about linguistic context pertain to whether aphasia disrupts receptive and expressive processing of discourse and text at microstructural and macrostructural levels. Traditionally, discourse and text comprehension is assessed clinically by presenting a paragraph and then asking a patient to answer questions about the content of the paragraph. Learning and recall components are unavoidable in such a task; and "online" processing, such as measuring saccadic eye movements during reading (e.g., Ehrlich and Rayner, 1983), has not yet been applied to studies of aphasia. Discourse is generally elicited by interviewing patients (e.g., Cicone, Wapner, Foldi, Zurif, and Gardner, 1979), or by asking them to describe a pictured situation (e.g., Yorkston and Beukelman, 1980) or tell a story portrayed in a series of pictures (e.g., Gleason et al., 1980).

Microstructure: Comprehension

What is the influence of aphasia on comprehension of coherence devices that connect sentences? Because articles are a coherence device, one suspicion is that the agrammatism of Broca's aphasia affects recognition of connections between sentences as well as production of a coherent sequence of ideas. An effect on comprehension is considered, because of the possible existence of "central agrammatism" underlying comprehension and production in Broca's aphasia (e.g., Berndt and Caramazza, 1980; Zurif, 1980). Research by Zurif and his colleagues has indicated that persons with Broca's aphasia become insensitive to semantic distinctions between "a or an" and "the" (e.g., Goodenough, Zurif, Weintraub, and Von Stockert, 1977). These functors distinguish between the first and second mention of a person or object or between new and given information, respectively. However, most research on receptive agrammatism has dealt with subject-object order rather than the uses of articles. More research on this question is needed.

Comprehension of coreference within a sentence was examined with statements such as 1a (Blumstein, Goodglass, Statlender, and Biber, 1983):

(1a) The boy watched the chef bandage himself.
(1b) The boy watching the chef bandaged himself.

Aphasic subjects displayed various levels of ability in comprehending the reflexive, depending on semantic and syntactic cues in a sentence. Minimal distance between the pronoun and its referent assisted the subjects, as the reflexive in 1b was more difficult than the reflexive in 1a. A paradigm for investigating referential coherence between sentences (Hirst and Brill, 1980) was applied in a study of persons with dementia (LeDoux, Blum, and Hirst, 1983). Two of five conditions are illustrated below:

(2a) John stood watching while Henry fell down some stairs.
(2b) He ran for a doctor.

(3a) John stood watching while Henry fell down some stairs.
(3b) He laughed with a vengeance.

Subjects were asked to choose whether the pronouns in 2b and 3b refer to John or Henry. Condition 2 had a strong bias to John, while condition 3 had a weak bias to John. A difference in choices between these conditions indicated that subjects were sensitive to strength of coreference.

Studies of the effect of context on comprehension have been common in investigations of aphasia. Among these studies are those that examine the effect of a preceding linguistic context on comprehension of a sentence. For example, Pierce and Beekman (1983) presented 4a as a context for 4b:

(4a) The woman has a book.
(4b) The woman went to the library.

Comprehension of 4b was tested by asking "Where did the woman go?" The link between such sentences was a common topic (i.e., reading material). Context facilitated comprehension of sentences such as 4b for low comprehending aphasic subjects. Evidently, the other subjects comprehended well enough so that contextual help was not needed for the sentence.

Microstructure: Expression

Expressive agrammatism can be shown to disrupt referential coherence between telegraphic sentences because of the omission of articles. With respect to examples 3 and 4 in Chapter 1, the following sequence is possible from a person with Broca's aphasia:

(5a) Bus. . . fast.
(5b) Bus. . . hit. . . girl.

In a conversation, it is most likely that the bus in 5b will be understood
to be the same as the bus in 5a. This is not certain, however; and if there
were two different buses, the patient could be misunderstood. One study
of agrammatism consisted of story completions to elicit article production
in at least three of 14 different grammatical constructions (Gleason,
Goodglass, Green, Ackerman, and Hyde, 1975). One type of story (e.g.,
6a) was designed to elicit declarative intransitive statements (e.g., 6b):

(6a) A baby has a toy. I take the toy away. What happens?
(6b) The baby cries.
(6c) "Baby cry."

The definite article in 6b signals reference back to the baby in 6a, while
a likely agrammatic response does not contain such a signal (e.g., 6c).
In Gleason's study, article omissions tended to be in the initial position.
Substitutions were rare, so that it is unlikely that someone with Broca's
aphasia will throw a listener off the track with "A baby cries." In fact,
Gleason's subjects occasionally substituted "He" for "The baby," a device
that, like "the," is also used for given information. Generally, researchers
have ignored such implications of article usage in agrammatism.

In discourse production, pronouns should be selected judiciously in
order to maintain referential coherence between sentences. Agrammatic
patients may omit pronouns, especially in the initial position of a phrase;
they may substitute an appropriate noun subject for an initial pronoun;
or they may change a pronoun, as from an expected "he" to "I" (Gleason
et al., 1975). Noun substitution appears to be a compensatory strategy
to ensure referential coherence, but pronoun changes would disrupt
coherence between utterances.

Kimbarow and Brookshire (1983) reported that nonfluent (e.g.,
Broca's) and fluent (e.g., anomic) aphasic subjects were careful about
ensuring that a listener knew the referent for pronouns used in descriptions
of one- and two-person video-recorded vignettes. With two-person
vignettes, pronoun reference was judged with respect to gender of
pronouns produced. Two-person vignettes could be more ambiguous in
terms of pronoun reference than one-person vignettes; reflecting their
sensitivity to this, subjects were better in describing two-person vignettes
than in describing one-person vignettes. While fluent subjects used an
expected excessive number of pronouns and their referent-to-pronoun ratio
was low, antecedents for the pronouns could still be identified in their
discourse. The investigators advocated paying attention to linguistic context

of numerous pronouns in the speech of fluent aphasic patients before making judgments about communicative adequacy simply based on the quantity of pronouns produced. The maintenance of referential coherence reflects an aphasic speaker's concern for taking the point of view of a listener, a sensitivity that contributes to distinguishing given and new information.

The jargon of Wernicke's aphasia is notorious for being "incoherent." Whether any of Kimbarow and Brookshire's (1983) fluent subjects included this syndrome is not clear from their discussion; however, it is doubtful that pronoun antecedents can be easily determined in neologistic jargon. In interviews with two such subjects, discourse consisted of incoherent shifts in semantic content across syntactic boundaries (Delis, Foldi, Hamby, Gardner, and Zurif, 1979).

Macrostructure: Comprehension

The ability to arrange printed sentences into a coherent story involves perceiving micro- and macrostructural relationships. Gardner and his Boston research group reported that aphasic subjects made as many sentence arrangement errors as persons with right hemisphere damage (Gardner, Brownell, Wapner, and Michelow, 1983). Both groups were impaired relative to normal controls. This result indicates that problems with sentence arrangement are not unique to aphasia. In another sentence arrangement study, global and Wernicke's patients had much more difficulty than Broca's and anomic patients; and anomic patients were unimpaired relative to normal controls (Huber and Gleber, 1982). Yet, the aphasic subjects in Gardner's study were equivalent to normals in number of sequencing errors with another task, namely, story retelling. Aphasic persons maintained narrative structure in one task but not in the other. The deficient performances may have been due to attributes of the sentence arrangement task. Consistent with Gardner's interpretation of other narrative limitations with aphasia, linguistic deficits in reading may interfere with realization of supposedly intact knowledge of narrative structure when arranging sentences.

One clinical method for addressing components of story structure draws upon the traditional paragraph comprehension format. Subsequent questions (or statements to verify) are used to examine a patient's sensitivity to (and recall of) themes and episodes. In research by Brookshire and Nicholas, themes were termed *main ideas*, and episodes were termed *details* (Brookshire and Nicholas, 1984; Wegner, Brookshire, and Nicholas, 1984). One test item was a story about two friends who got into a fight at a bar and then wound up in jail and before a judge the next morning. A statement to verify about a main idea (i.e., theme) was "Two men were at a bar"; and a statement about a detail (i.e., episode) was "The bartender called the cops." These sentences concerned information stated directly in the paragraph, while *indirectly stated* themes and episodes were represented with sentences about information that could be inferred from what was said. Intersentential information was tested by virtue of the consistent reference to a main idea that occurs throughout a coherent paragraph.

If Brookshire and Nicholas' subjects were sensitive to such repeated reference, then main ideas should have been recalled more accurately than details. With auditory presentation, aphasic subjects comprehended main ideas better than details; and directness made no difference (Brookshire and Nicholas, 1984). Wapner, Hamby, and Gardner (1981) indicated that their aphasic subjects reported the main point or moral of stories when they could. Gardner concluded that "in the face of reduced production or comprehension, what resources are available to these subjects are devoted to central information" (Gardner et al., 1983, p. 182).

The macrostructural level may be involved in the studies of sentence comprehension with a preceding context. Instead of a preceding sentence, as in Pierce and Beekman's study (1983) mentioned earlier, the prior context may be a paragraph. Nicholas and Brookshire (1983) examined comprehension of comparative and embedded clause statements (e.g., 7b) with and without prior narrative context that is shown in 7a:

> (7a) School was over and several children were standing in line waiting for the school bus. Three girls were at the front of the line, talking and laughing. Suddenly, a boy ran up and pushed one of the girls out of the line.
> (7b) The girl pushed by the boy was eating an apple.

Narrative context facilitated comprehension of embedded clause sentences for nonfluent aphasic subjects. It was of no help for comparative statements and fluent aphasic subjects.

Such effects may depend on a number of factors, such as the nature of cohesion between a test sentence and its prior context, and the kind of information requested among picture choices used to test sentence comprehension. Nicholas and Brookshire (1983) expressed a need to determine the components of context that are facilitative and those that are not helpful. For example, the test sentence may possess common reference with only the preceding sentence or with several sentences. The common reference may be necessary to understand the test sentence, or it may only provide repetitive exposure to a linguistic unit. Type of microstructural cohesion device may make a difference. In such prior context studies, narrative may only define the length of context, but not the structural components that *must* be processed by the subject in order to make an accurate response.

Macrostructure: Expression

Narrative discourse often is elicited with picture-story sequences and and story-retelling tasks. Agrammatism of nonfluent aphasia can make a story line difficult to discern (Rivers and Love, 1980). Using both procedures, Ulatowska and her colleagues have examined varied aphasias with moderate degree of impairment (Ulatowska, North, and Macaluso-Haynes, 1981; Ulatowska, Freedman-Stern, Doyel, Macaluso-Haynes, and North, 1983). While aphasic subjects were rated lower than normal subjects in overall clarity of narrative production, aphasic subjects tended to maintain the sequence of elements in a story as if they retained knowledge of narrative schemas. Differences from normal occurred with respect to quantity of element production, especially in a reduced number of setting, resolution, and evaluation clauses. Aphasic subjects were unimpaired in terms of number of action clauses produced. Severely impaired subjects, on the other hand, appeared to retain the intent to tell stories but could not produce the elements of discourse (Bond, Ulatowska, Macaluso-Haynes, and May, 1983). Ulatowska also has found that moderately impaired aphasic persons are able to produce the essential elements of "procedural" discourse, which is instruction on how to do something (Ulatowska, Doyel, Stern, Haynes, and North, 1983). Ulatowska and Gardner appear to agree that moderately and mildly impaired aphasic persons retain a sense for narrative structure that is often masked by linguistic deficit (Gardner et al., 1983).

PARALINGUISTIC CONTEXT: PROSODY

Some prosodic devices have been manipulated in stimuli to facilitate receptive processing by aphasic persons. These features have not been studied frequently as communicative devices per se and, therefore, have been ignored in clinical assessment of aphasia. With respect to verbal expression, impaired prosody has been associated with nonfluent or Broca's aphasia, and somewhat normal prosody has been attributed to fluent aphasias.

Emotion

The neurology of emotion has been investigated in terms of whether the cerebral hemispheres differ in their responsibility for this behavior (e.g.,

Bear, 1983; Bryden, 1982) and whether impairment of emotion is a feature of right hemisphere brain damage (e.g., Ross, 1981; Tucker, Watson, and Heilman, 1977). Aphasic persons, on the other hand, are often characterized as possessing a relatively normal range of emotional capability.

Recognition of emotion conveyed with prosody has been studied by comparing subjects' judgments about sad, angry, happy, and neutral sounding utterances. Because semantic content may also convey emotional state (e.g., "I am sad"), the influence of linguistic information usually is minimized by presenting semantically "neutral" statements (e.g., "I am here") that are colored by different prosodic hues. Patients are asked to choose among pictured faces expressing these emotions. Aphasic subjects have displayed deficits in recognition of emotion through prosody, comparable to right hemisphere damaged subjects (Schlanger, Schlanger, and Gerstman, 1976). In the study by Schlanger and coworkers, high-verbal aphasic subjects were still 77 per cent correct, compared to 70 per cent with right hemisphere damage.

In other research, aphasic persons were better than right hemisphere damaged persons and relatively close to normals in comprehending emotional prosody (Heilman, Bowers, Speedie, and Coslett, 1984; Tucker et al., 1977). In Heilman's research, he tended to use only conduction aphasic subjects, as opposed to the general aphasic group in the study by Schlangers and colleagues. Also, the composition of Heilman's right hemisphere damaged group was different. Nevertheless, further research has shown that performance of aphasic persons may be maximized when prosodic contour and semantic content coincide (Seron, Van Der Kaa, Van Der Linden, Remitz, and Feyereisen, 1982).

Expression of emotion through prosody has not been studied with aphasic subjects, as it has been with right hemisphere damaged persons. For example, Tucker and coworkers (1977) chose not to test aphasic controls with an imitative task, because their deficit in verbal expression would not permit prosodic capacity to be expressed. Danly and Shapiro (1982) studied the mechanics of certain elements of prosody, finding some strengths and weaknesses in Broca's aphasia and finding an occasional "hypermelodic" quality in Wernicke's aphasia (Danly, Cooper, and Shapiro, 1983).

Semantics and Syntax

The most severely impaired aphasic persons are able to respond as if they recognize whether an utterance is a statement, question, or command (Green and Boller, 1974), and one explanation is that these patients perceive paralinguistic cues to speaker intentions or speech acts. Heilman and his colleagues (1984) studied recognition of prosody in declarative, interrogative, and imperative sentences by filtering out the semantic content. Subjects identified form by pointing to the appropriate punctuation mark. Aphasic subjects displayed deficits that equalled a right hemisphere damaged group. Heilman concluded that aphasia disrupts the semantic or syntactic use of paralinguistic context to a much greater degree (or more often) than it disrupts the use of prosody to recognize emotion.

Patients with Broca's aphasia were studied with respect to recognition of stress (8a,b) and juncture (9a,b) cues to the deep structure and phrasing of ambiguous sentences (Baum, Daniloff, Daniloff, and Lewis, 1982):

(8a) They fed her *dog* biscuits.
(8b) They fed her dog *biscuits*.

(9a) He noticed its nose here.
(9b) He noticed it snows here.

The aphasic group was deficient in processing both cues, but this problem was related to severity of Broca's aphasia. Less severely impaired subjects had near-normal scores. The investigators, however, also concluded that a deficit with paralinguistic cues still exists in patients who perform well on standard clinical tests of comprehension.

Pashek and Brookshire (1982) examined the effect of lexical stress on paragraph comprehension by aphasic subjects. They found that exaggerated stress on a crucial word within a sentence was of assistance in improving accuracy of answering questions about the paragraphs. However, such stress appears to have served no particular communicative function itself, such as conveying emotion or signaling new information. It would be of interest to determine whether aphasic persons are sensitive to appropriate and inappropriate placement of stress relative to new and old information, respectively, within a paragraph.

Paralinguistic devices also signal semantic distinctions for lexical units, especially in the so-called tonal languages. For example, in the Thai language, a particular phoneme combination can mean "to be stuck," "a kind of spice," "to kill," or "leg" depending on pitch variation; and aphasic speakers of this language are impaired in comprehending such distinctions (Gandour and Dardarananda, 1983). In English, syllabic stress may be necessary to identify whether "convict" is a noun or a verb. Stress and juncture differentiate "sorehead" from "sore head." In a task that was difficult for normal controls, Blumstein and Goodglass (1972) concluded that aphasic persons can make such distinctions. Of course, the only time such utterances would appear in isolation, thereby depending on help solely from paralinguistic conventions, would be in a study or clinical assessment of prosodic abilities. Usually other contexts would be available to assist in disambiguation.

EXTRALINGUISTIC CONTEXT

Now we consider the aphasic person's ability to utilize contexts outside of language and its prosodic trappings. We shall deal with recognition and generation of these contexts, and we shall discuss some of the interactions between extralinguistic contexts and disordered language performance. As we said in Chapter 1, extralinguistic contexts are the ones that are most commonly associated with pragmatic considerations.

Setting

Clinical observation indicates that aphasic individuals generally are well-oriented to situations in which a conversation might occur; they recognize people, places, and things. This orientation enables them to use their environment in order to communicate their ideas and their wishes. Foldi, Cicone, and Gardner (1983) introduced their chapter on pragmatics with a vignette involving "Mr. Harvey," a hospitalized patient who pointed to a medical chart rack in a ward office in order to convey his need to take his chart to an afternoon appointment with an ophthalmologist. Aphasic persons, at least, will point to people, places, and things (e.g., Holland, 1982).

Patients' ability to recognize settings may be anticipated with a look at how well they process components of situations through single modalites. Studies with a variety of nonverbal tasks presented by Cohen and Kelter in Germany are of interest in this regard. While we shall be pointing out areas of deficiency, according to comparisons with superior control groups, performances of aphasic persons on these tasks still are good relative to their scores on language tasks. Often the weakest performance hovers around 80 per cent correct, even for severely impaired aphasic subjects. This level has been observed in matching familiar sounds to their source, although persons with Wernicke's aphasia may be below this level (Cohen, Kelter, and Woll, 1980; Faglioni, Spinnler, and Vignolo, 1969; Spinnler and Vignolo, 1966). The recognition of environmental sounds appears to be closely related to severity of auditory language comprehension deficit. Levels of about 88 per cent accuracy have been found in associating colors with line drawings of objects (Basso, Faglioni, and Spinnler, 1976; Cohen and Kelter, 1979; Cohen et al., 1980). There is also some difficulty in matching objects according to common attributes

(Kelter, Cohen, Engel, List, and Strohner, 1977). Cohen and coworkers (1980) reviewed evidence indicating that these problems may not be related to perceptual deficit but, instead, may be due to dysfunction at the conceptual or "preverbal" level of cognition.

Cohen and Kelter conducted more specific comparisons of picture matching according to similarities in attributes, function, action, and situations. With weakest scores approaching 80 per cent accuracy, the scores of aphasic persons were above 90 per cent in relating objects based on situational characteristics, as in choosing from "guitar" and "violin" the object that goes best with "bullfight." Situational judgments were the only conditions in which both Wernicke's and Broca's aphasic persons were comparable to brain-injured nonaphasic controls, indicating that "analytical isolation, identification, and conceptual comparison of highly specific individual aspects" is a feature of aphasia (Cohen et al., 1980, p. 343).

As indicated in Cohen and Kelter's research, aphasic persons have mild problems in detailed conceptual comparisons, but they do quite well in recognizing global characteristics of situations. They recognized emotion in pictured situations, as in a person being mugged (Cicone, Wapner, and Gardner, 1980); and they recognized humor conveyed visually in cartoons (Gardner, Ling, Flamm, and Silverman, 1975). However, when connecting a series of episodes in a story, subjects with global and Wernicke's aphasia (i.e., severe language comprehension deficit) were worse than other aphasic subjects in arranging pictures into a logical sequence (Huber and Gleber, 1982). Broca's and anomic aphasic subjects approached the level of normal control subjects in arranging pictured episodes of a story.

While most studies of language comprehension and production in aphasia involve pictured "settings" either to point to or to describe, a few studies have dealt with the effect of the presence of such context on comprehension ability. In a study mentioned previously in this chapter, Pierce and Beekman (1983) presented a picture that was analogous to the prior sentence context of 4a. The picture aided comprehension of a sentence by low comprehending subjects, as measured by answers to questions about the sentence. Therefore, a simple context (e.g., "The boy is dirty") may help a person with Wernicke's aphasia comprehend "The boy was playing in the mud," when asked "Where was the boy playing?" and given a choice of pointing to mud or a pool. In another study, paragraph reading was improved by prior presentation of a picture related to content of the paragraph (Waller and Darley, 1978). Aphasic persons comprehend language a little better in the presence of relevant extralinguistic context than without such context.

In addition to pictures, real objects are used as props in the clinical observation of language behavior, especially when employing the "following instructions" paradigm for assessing language comprehension. Real objects may be considered to be contextual information that influences language comprehension, as indicated by the fact that, in developing the Token Test, DeRenzi and Vignolo (1962) rejected the use of real objects in an instruction-following task so that language comprehension could be tested as purely as possible. There have been mixed findings as to whether the use of real objects in a Token Test format actually exerts a favorable influence on comprehension scores (Kreindler, Gheorghita, and Voinescu, 1971; Lesser, 1979; Lohman and Prescott, 1978; Martino, Pizzamiglio, and Razzano, 1976). However, Seron and Deloche (1981) showed how props can influence an aphasic person's response to prepositions. The influence stems from the plausibility of spatial relationships between particular objects. That is, a coin is more likely to be placed "in" a money box rather that "on" it. Persons with Broca's aphasia were more accurate following instructions when a preposition was congruent with the contextual bias created by props than when a preposition and props were incongruent.

Lubinski (1981a, 1981b) has described circumstances in which a setting itself may be "impaired" with respect to promoting maximal communication. She called such settings the "communication-impaired environment" and associated them particularly with some institutional settings. An impaired environment would contain restrictions on talking, negative or prejudicial attitudes toward certain interactions, poor lighting and acoustics, and large numbers of persons who are communicatively impaired in one way or another.

Participants: Internal and External Contexts

As indicated in Chapter 1, the participant factor provides internal and external contexts. This distinction is particularly important when the aphasic person is the center of our attention in a conversational dyad. He or she possesses internal contexts such as prior knowledge and emotional state and external contexts such as his or her own movements. Additional external contexts with respect to an aphasic participant include the other person in a dyad, with his or her own conceptual knowledge, emotional state, and movements. Therefore, our discussion of shared knowlege, for example, will pertain to an aphasic person's internal and external contexts.

Shared Knowledge. One method for studying the influence of a patient's own conceptual knowledge on language comprehension involves manipulating the semantic *plausibility* of a sentence. The finding that nonreversible sentences are sometimes easier to comprehend than reversible statements has been explained with the notion that aphasic persons, especially those with Broca's aphasia, realize that confusing subjects in a nonreversible sentence (e.g., 10) would produce an impossible or implausible event (Caramazza and Zurif, 1976):

(10) The *apple* that the *boy* is eating is red.

Persons with aphasia find comprehension easier when statements fit their understanding of the world (e.g., 11a) than when statements refer to less likely events (e.g., 11b) (Deloche and Seron, 1981; Heilman and Scholes, 1976; Heeschen, 1980):

(11a) The patient calls the nurse.
(11b) The thief arrests the policeman.

The difference between such statements has been greater in Broca's aphasia than in Wernicke's aphasia in some studies, a finding that is similar to Seron and Deloche's (1981) results in studying the plausibility of congruence between prepositions and props. However, Kudo (1984) found that more plausible statements were easier to comprehend for all major types of aphasia. One study in which plausibility had no effect consisted of statements such as the following (Goodglass et al., 1979):

(12a) The man greeted by his wife was smoking a pipe.
(12b) The woman greeting her husband was smoking a pipe.

The implausible statement (12b) may have been unlikely, in traditional circles, rather than impossible. Either the plausibility effect is inconsistent or some subjects have different knowledge bases in which 12b is as likely to occur as 12a. Most studies indicate that knowledge affects comprehension, which has led developers of aphasia tests to use content that is assumed to be well known by everyone.

Some research has indicated that the conceptual knowledge (i.e., *semantic memory*) of persons with Wernicke's aphasia might be somewhat shaky. While Cohen and Kelter suggested that analysis of details might be reduced in all aphasias, others have suggested that the static structure of semantic memory might have become disorganized, especially in patients who have posterior brain damage with poor auditory comprehension. A variety of nonverbal and verbal tasks have revealed differences in association and concept comparison strategies (Grober, Perecman, Kellar, and Brown, 1980; Grossman, 1978, 1981; Semenza, Denes, Lucchese, and Bisiacchi, 1980). These problems may be a result of disrupted analytical strategies with intact conceptual knowledge or changes in conceptual knowledge itself. Clinicians should look out for resolution of this matter, because treatment might be directed toward an impairment of internal context as well as toward language.

Dealing with other conversational participants begins with recognizing who they are. Recognizing a person's identity is essential for meaningful communication, so that appropriate prior knowledge can be activated and appropriate assumptions about that person's point of view can be invoked in relying on the cooperative principle. Face recognition has been studied frequently relative to asymmetry of brain function (e.g., Bryden, 1982). Because the right hemisphere has been shown to be better than the left at recognizing unfamiliar faces (Levy, Trevarthen, and Sperry, 1972) and familiar faces (Levin and Koch-Weser, 1982), this ability may be spared when the left hemisphere is damaged. Difficulties with face recognition can occur from brain damage, as shown in cases of dementia (Cummings and Benson, 1983) and focal lesions of the right hemisphere (e.g., Cicone et al., 1980; Dekosky, Heilman, Bowers, and Valenstein, 1980). In a face matching task, Cicone's aphasic subjects were better than subjects with right hemisphere damage; and, of the aphasic group, only the subjects who had anterior brain damage showed some difficulty (still 91 per cent correct). Dekosky and coworkers found aphasic persons to be equivalent to normal adults in recognizing unfamiliar faces.

Knowledge that is shared between an aphasic individual and others in a communicative interaction is necessary for communication to occur most accurately and efficiently. In Foldi's vignette mentioned earlier, one nurse was not able to understand what Mr. Harvey meant when he pointed to the chart rack (Foldi et al., 1983). However, another nurse knew what he meant, because she remembered his afternoon appointment and his need to take his chart with him. The second nurse's knowledge contributed to the effectiveness of Mr. Harvey's gestured communication. Clinicians realize that communicative difficulties in early contacts with an aphasic patient are caused, in part, by lack of knowledge of the patient and of the patient's chosen topic. Clients with most types of communicative disorders are often evaluated by unfamiliar clinicians after weeks of treatment, because clinicians know that increased familiarity has changed the communicative situation from what it was during the first week or two of treatment. The knowledgeable nurse and Mr. Harvey underscore a point made in Chapter 1, namely, that communicative success depends on knowledge shared by the clinician and client, as well as on the client's linguistic abilities.

Emotional State. This internal context is discussed with respect to whether aphasic persons possess normal emotional arousal. One method employed to infer emotional response is to measure physiological components of arousal such as skin resistance, heart rate, and respiration. In one study, galvanic skin response (GSR) was measured during tactile stimulation of brain damaged subjects (Heilman, Schwartz, and Watson, 1978). While right hemisphere damaged subjects had a reduced GSR relative to normal controls, aphasic subjects had a higher GSR relative to normals. Responses of brain damaged subjects to neutral and emotional picture stimuli were measured by Morrow, Vrtunski, Kim, and Boller (1981) with a polygraph device that records GSR and respiration. Left hemisphere damaged subjects displayed less physiological arousal than normal controls. However, like the normal group, these brain injured subjects experienced enhanced arousal to emotional stimuli relative to neutral stimuli. A right hemisphere damaged group, on the other hand, showed less arousal than the left hemisphere group and no difference between neutral and emotional stimuli. In another study, the appropriateness of aphasic arousal was indicated behaviorally by their "mirth" responses to humor in cartoons (Gardner, Ling, Flamm, et al., 1975). Aphasic subjects' facial expressions in response to pictures indicated that emotional response was usually accurate and, in some cases, was more expressive than in normal subjects (Buck and Duffy, 1980).

The emotional state in aphasic persons may consist of two abnormal factors: (a) occasional disinhibition of appropriate arousal in some cases, and (b) psychological reactions and adjustments to the loss of language and motor functions. The former has been referred to as emotional lability (Eisenson, 1984). Gainotti (1972) found that left brain-damaged subjects were characterized by catastrophic and anxious-depressive reactions, while right brain-damaged subjects tended to be indifferent. The heightened arousal to tactile vibration in Heilman's study may be indicative of some disinhibition. The emotional behavior of aphasic persons, however, may not be indicative of a special impairment of emotion caused by brain damage but, instead, may reflect natural psychological response to the loss of function and the frustration from disability imposed by brain damage (Bryden, 1982). The only exception would be those with Wernicke's aphasia, who do not seem to be aware of their disorder and present a euphoric pattern of behavior (Sparks, 1978). Persons with nonfluent aphasia in general appear to be more depressed than those with fluent aphasia several months after onset (Robinson and Benson, 1981).

Language-context interactions regarding emotional arousal may have special implications for aphasic persons. Emotional content in language may evoke improved language performance, possibly as a result of help from the right cerebral hemisphere. In a study of normal male adults, response to visual hemifield presentation of emotional words (e.g., kill, love, rape) appeared to involve the right hemisphere more than nonemotional words (e.g., time, fact, span) (Graves, Landis, and Goodglass, 1981). Severely impaired aphasic patients were more responsive to sentences with emotional content than sentences with neutral content (Boller, Cole, Vrtunski, Patterson, and Kim, 1979). Affective content enhanced recognition of emotion conveyed in sentences above levels achieved with prosodic cues alone (Seron et al., 1982). It is possible that emotional arousal enhances linguistic performance in aphasic persons, a question that still needs to be investigated more directly.

Participants' Role. Role can be manipulated easily in a communicative interaction with an aphasic client. Differences in role are accompanied by differences in knowledge of a topic; and role differences between two participants in a conversational dyad bring differences in shared knowlege to bear on communication. A few comparisons of role differences have been attempted with a small number of subjects. Familiarity has been a primary consideration, as aphasic individuals have been paired with familiar adults (spouses, clinicians) and unfamiliar clinicians or strangers (Gurland, Chwat, and Wollner, 1982; Larkins and Webster, 1981; Lubinski et al., 1980). Yorkston, Beukelman, and Flowers (1980) compared experienced and inexperienced clinicians as communicative partners. Lubinski and coworkers (1980) observed that the different "agendas" of the spouse and clinician affected the occurrence of miscommunications and repairs of these "breakdowns." Because shared knowledge is a powerful variable in the pairing of conversational partners, it is possible that the effect of semantic plausibility is suggestive of effects that might be seen when an aphasic parnter converses with other partners in different roles.

Movement. This extralinguistic context is generated by the aphasic person and by his or her communication partners. Identifying communicative assets and deficits with this context depends on the type of movement that is considered. Differentiated movements (e.g., limb gestures) can be defined according to their characteristics, such as simple (single position) or complex (sequence of positions). They can also be defined according to their functional level, such as propositional or subpropositional. Terminology can be confusing when comparing studies of the same behavior. Numerous contrasts have appeared in the aphasia literature (e.g., symbolic-nonsymbolic, referential-nonreferential, propositional-subpropositional, iconic-noniconic, and transitive-intransitive). Different authors using different terms have produced some inconsistency of definition, such as "iconic" being a classification that is separate from "symbolic" (Peterson and Kirshner, 1981) and being a subcategory of "referential" (Cicone et al., 1979). Our classification of gestures appears in Chapter 3.

In this segment, we are primarily interested in gestures as they are used by patients in conversations, as opposed to the same gestures being elicited in clinical tests. Let us consider four conversations involving two Broca's and two Wernicke's aphasic subjects being interviewed by an experimenter (Cicone et al., 1979). Cicone found that general features of gesturing corresponded to verbal patterns of the nonfluent and fluent aphasic subjects, a correspondence that was subsequently recognized by Duffy, Duffy, and Mercaitis (1984) as well. In Cicone's study, there was a greater-than-normal frequency, complexity, and ambiguity of gesturing with Wernicke's aphasia; and there was a reduced frequency and complexity of gesturing with Broca's aphasia. Both types of aphasia produced pantomime for around 38 per cent of their "information-carrying" gestures. Subjects with Broca's aphasia used emblems (i.e., conventional gestures) for 22 per cent of their gestures, while those with Wernicke's aphasia did not use emblems at all. Those with Broca's aphasia also did a little writing in the air, displaying of numbers, and pointing to present objects.

The subjects with Wernicke's aphasia also produced what Cicone and coworkers (1979) described as pointing to an area in space in association with a verbal reference. These general movements were produced to the same extent as pantomime. These severely impaired fluent subjects either used pantomime or were vague in their gesturing. These subjects displayed another feature of gesturing that was related to the deficient coherence of their verbal expression (Delis et al., 1979). That is, normal control subjects produced semantically coherent embedded clauses during their interviews, without a tendency to gesture at the beginning of these clauses. The two subjects with Wernicke's aphasia tended to gesture at the beginning of their numerous semantically discontinuous embedded clauses. Therefore, these subjects may have used a few of their gestures to signal shifts of semantic intentions.

In another study of free conversation, 92 per cent of all gestures in fluent and nonfluent aphasias were designated as gesticulations (Goldblum, cited in Feyereisen and Seron, 1982a). Cicone and coworkers (1979), on the other hand, recorded 82 per cent of all gestures with Broca's aphasia as being "referential" and 59 per cent with Wernicke's aphasia as being referential. Cicone defined referential to include symbols and some signals, but this category excluded gesticulation. Goldblum saw most movements as being gesticulations, and Cicone saw most movements as being referential. This dramatic difference between observations could be a result of differences in definition, subjects, conditions, and scoring method. Therefore, generalizations are not possible based on this research, and the clinician should simply take note of the presence or absence of all types of gesture in conversation with a patient. According to Cicone, from only four subjects, aphasic persons have the capacity and inclination to produce some symbolic gestures, usually of the iconic variety (i.e., pantomime), during conversation. He suggested that these subjects did not capitalize on their full potential for producing symbolic movements.

CAPABILITIES WITH THE GESTURE MODE

While the full potential for gestural expression may not be forthcoming in an interview or in natural conversation, this potential may be seen when specific gestures are elicited with clinical tasks such as imitation and following instructions. This section is intended to review clinical studies in which the gestural modality, receptive and expressive, has been observed in isolation, that is, without situational contexts or accompanying verbal behavior. There has been considerable interest in nonverbal abilities that would augment or replace a limited linguistic system in order to improve communicative ability. However, several investigators have revealed that there are limitations in the gestural mode, primarily with one type of gesture, namely, pantomime.

A number of clinical aphasiologists have been curious about whether or not pantomime deficit stems from a general symbolic impairment (i.e., *asymbolia*) that also produces the linguistic deficits of aphasia. The issue of whether gesture deficit and language deficit stem from the same cognitive deficit is important to the clinician, because a resolution will influence approach and prognosis in attempting to change gestural behavior. Sensitivity to the variety of gestures is also important (see Chapter 3), because conclusions about pantomime may not necessarily apply to other forms of gestural behavior.

Facial Gesture: Recognition and Expression

Aphasic adults should have little difficulty recognizing facial expressions as signals to emotional state, because the right hemisphere appears to be primarily responsible for recognizing emotion in facial expression (Ley and Bryden, 1979). They have been superior to subjects with right hemisphere damage in recognizing emotional expression in faces, but they have been mildly deficient in comparison to normal adults. In one study, aphasic subjects matched emotional expressions at 85 per cent accuracy (Cicone et al., 1980); but, in another study, they were equivalent to normal subjects in discriminating emotional faces (Dekosky et al., 1980). Recognition of facial expression has not been studied as often with aphasic subjects as it has been with normal adults and people with right hemisphere brain damage. Our clinical experience is that aphasic adults recognize the meaning of facial expressions; but research indicates that some patients, perhaps according to type or severity, may experience some minor confusions about the meaning of a facial gesture.

Buck and Duffy (1980) examined facial expressions of aphasic subjects in a study that included a "new information condition" as discussed in the first chapter. Subjects were shown color slides representing familiar people, pleasant scenes, unpleasant scenes, and unusual photographic effects. Instead of evaluating facial responses as they occurred, the experimenters recorded subjects' facial expressions on videotape and then played them back to "receivers" who did not know exactly what slides had been seen. The independent observers guessed, from each facial expression, the type of slide that the subjects had been viewing. The accuracy of the receivers' guesses was taken as a measure of the subjects' accuracy in emotional facial expression. While accuracy scores were generally low for all subject groups, reflecting the subjectivity of the measure, aphasic subjects were more accurate than normal controls and much more accurate than subjects with right hemisphere damage. It would appear that aphasic persons are not deficient in facial expression when it is an affective display. Duffy and Buck (1979) concluded that subpropositional gesture is intact with aphasia and that, in some cases, aphasic individuals fail to inhibit reactions to emotional stimuli.

Some aphasic persons have a mild right facial paresis that will inhibit or distort propositional and subpropositional facial expression. While this motor disorder may not be severe enough to prohibit meaningful facial expression, psychological reaction to this change in appearance may lead to self-conscious monitoring of facial expression. We knew one aphasic individual who would refrain from smiling when greeting people, because he did not want to reveal a distorted expression. This example demontrates a need for assisting the patient in psychological adjustment that may lead to improvements of simple pragmatic nonverbal communicative functions.

Limb Gesture: Recognition

Of the many types of gesture, pantomime has been the most frequently studied with respect to recognition ability. The receptive mode has been studied for the purpose of identifying the presence of asymbolia, so that motor disorders would not interfere with observation of this possible cognitive deficit. Pantomime recognition has also been studied with respect to cerebral localization of this function (Ferro, Martins, Mariano, and Castro-Caldas, 1983). This ability is usually tested by requiring clients to match a gesture with a pictured object that is appropriate to the meaning of the gesture.

Some disagreement exists as to whether aphasia is necessarily accompanied by a deficit in pantomime recognition. Different analyses have led to somewhat different conclusions. For example, recognition deficit appears to characterize the aphasia population as a whole when considering average group performance and statistical difference from normal controls (Duffy, Duffy, and Pearson, 1975). Further evidence for the existence of asymbolia has come from strong correlations between pantomime recognition deficit and linguistic deficits (Duffy and Duffy, 1981), especially between pantomime deficit and receptive language deficit (e.g., Ferro, Santos, Castro-Caldas, and Mariano, 1980). However, when the number of subjects falling below a cut-off score (the floor of a normal range) is determined, recognition deficit does not appear to be an inherent feature of aphasia. The proportion of aphasic adults showing deficits in this way varies from 41 to 74 per cent (Gainotti and Lemmo, 1976; Seron, Van Der Kaa, Remitz, and Van Der Linden, 1979; Varney, 1982). Some studies have shown no relationship between gesture recognition and severity of aphasia (Daniloff, Noll, Fristoe, and Lloyd, 1982; Feyereisen and Seron, 1982b; Seron et al., 1979). Others have found a weak relationship between pantomime recognition and auditory language comprehension (Gainotti and Lemmo, 1976). While a relationship has been observed between pantomime recognition and reading deficits, some subjects with aphasia had a reading deficit without pantomime recognition impairment (Varney, 1978). Therefore, pantomime recognition deficit may not be a component of symbolic impairment in some people; and Ferro and coworkers (1980) concluded that the presence of this deficit depends on the type of aphasia, that is, it is related to global aphasia but not to Wernicke's aphasia.

Because pantomime recognition deficit does occur in some cases of aphasia, it has been of interest to determine whether patients respond in ways that are similar to responses in tests of word recognition. For example, when response choices are pictures that are semantically similar, word recognition is less accurate than when pictures are unrelated. Duffy and Watkins (1984) found that pantomime recognition accuracy was negatively influenced by semantic similarity among picture choices and that this effect was related to the effect of semantic relatedness on a word recognition test. Duffy and Watkins concluded that this semantic dimension of pantomime recognition provides more evidence for the existence of asymbolia. Varney and Benton (1982) observed a strong tendency for errors to be semantically related pictures, which they interpreted as reflecting partial or vague comprehension of pantomimes when errors do occur.

By utilizing a unique manner of controlling picture choices, Seron and coworkers (1979) offered an analysis of pantomime recognition that provides an additional insight into this mode of communication. Besides providing a semantic foil in the set of picture choices, they included a "morphological" foil, which was an object that could be manipulated similarly to the target object (but was not semantically related). For example, a picture of a person miming the playing of a piano was presented; and among the picture choices were the target (piano), a semantic foil (harp), and a morphological foil (desk). Of the errors made by aphasic subjects, morphological choices were as likely to occur as semantic choices. Therefore, when a pantomime must be recognized without a meaningful context to resolve ambiguities, the gesture could look like something entirely different from what was intended.

Pantomime and other gestures still appear to be a major remaining source of information for the aphasic individual, because recognition levels usually remain high in spite of statistical differences from normal that are indicative of a "deficit." The average proportion that were correct in Duffy and Duffy's (1981) study was 87 per cent. A substantial proportion of aphasic subjects has been within normal range in other studies, including 59 per cent (Varney, 1982), 38 per cent (Gainotti and Lemmo, 1976), and 26 per cent (Seron et al., 1979). Fourteen subjects averaged 22 of 24 correct in recognizing symbols of Amer-Ind code (Daniloff et al., 1982). Therefore, aphasic individuals are likely to be aided in receiving messages by watching gestures that accompany speech or occur alone. In fact, persons with right hemiplegia (two thirds clearly with aphasia) scored higher on pegboard tasks by following pantomimed commands than by following oral commands, while the reverse was seen for patients with left hemiplegia (Fordyce and Jones, 1966). Furthermore, severely impaired aphasic adults performed simple object manipulations and body movements better when instructions included a combination of pantomime and speech than when either mode was used by itself (Beukelman, Yorkston, and Waugh, 1980). Pantomime recognition may be intact in some aphasic patients; and, when it is deficient in others, it is likely to be a mild deficiency with some misinterpretation occurring because a pantomime out of context can be somewhat ambiguous anyway.

Limb Gesture: Expression

Clinical expectations from this mode should be tempered with the realization that gestures vary widely in their intentionality and symbolic nature and that expressive deficits occur in select contexts and for different reasons. Patients with anterior unilateral brain damage are likely to have a hemiplegia interfering with use of one limb. Either limb apraxia or asymbolia would be exhibited bilaterally in fluent aphasias and unilaterally (usually the left side) in nonfluent aphasias.

Limb Apraxia. Limb apraxia is an inability to perform an action on command, when the same action can be performed spontaneously with natural motivation and context. A typical example is the patient who fails to light a cigarette when instructed to do so and then five minutes later, when wanting to smoke, lights a cigarette quite naturally. It is often missed outside the clinic because ". . . neither the patient nor the patient's relatives call the physician's attention to a disorder that in the great majority of cases only appears in the testing situation and does not trouble the patient in everyday life" (DeRenzi, Motti, and Nichelli, 1980, p. 9).

Identification of limb apraxia can be tricky, especially because there may be two versions of the disorder, namely, ideomotor apraxia (IMA) and ideational apraxia (IA). Various attempts have been made to establish these versions as two distinct disorders based on complexity of movement and whether a gesture is made with or without objects (DeRenzi, Pieczuro, and Vignolo, 1968; Heilman, 1973). There has been a tendency to test IMA with imitation (involving short-term memory of a movement) and IA with following commands (supposedly involving "recall" of a movement from long-term memory). Instead of attempting to resolve the mysteries swirling around the variations of limb apraxia, we shall focus on the performance of aphasic persons on tests of limb apraxia.

Imitation is an early stage for training gestures in severely impaired aphasic patients (Helm-Estabrooks, Fitzpatrick, and Barresi, 1982). Most patients are impaired when tested on the imitation of simple and complex symbolic and nonsymbolic gestures (DeRenzi et al., 1968, 1980). In a test of imitating "simple and complex, transitive and intransitive" gestures (Duffy and Duffy, 1981), aphasic subjects averaged a lower score (16.1) than normal controls (18.7). The range for aphasic subjects (8.2 to 19.7) indicated that many scored within the normal range (18.0 to 19.6). These tasks, especially in DeRenzi's studies, consisted of conventiona', intransitive gestures (i.e., emblems). As DeRenzi suggested, natural production of the victory sign, a salute, or crossing oneself may often be normal. However, many studies of imitative ability do not include direct observation of more natural performance of the gestures that are imitated.

When patients are asked to *follow commands*, investigators control for deficits of auditory comprehension, so that scores may be valid measures of motor function. Therefore, patients tend not to be instructed to "show me the victory sign," but instead are asked to demonstrate the use of common objects with the objects present. DeRenzi and coworkers

(1968) found that 66 per cent of their aphasic subjects were not impaired in performing indicative movements with such objects. Their test was similar to subtests II and III of the *Porch Index of Communicative Ability* (Porch, 1981). Few aphasic persons appear to be completely successful with these subtests. Fourteen per cent attained 13.00 or better on subtest III when a score of 16.00 is the maximum level of performance (Porch, 1967). Average performance on this subtest was 11.40 (Porch, 1981). However, normal adults averaged 12.79 on subtest III (Duffy, Keith, Shane, and Podraza, 1976). Therefore, with respect to normal indicative movements, aphasic performance may not be much different on average. Nevertheless, limb apraxia occurs frequently with aphasia, because there is an anatomical contiguity between premotor and language areas of the left hemisphere.

Asymbolia. With an absence of motor impairment, an aphasic person still may have difficulty producing pantomimes that are illustrations of object use without the object present. Pantomime has been studied more often than emblems in a propositional format. Nevertheless, impaired propositional production of emblems has been observed also (Duffy and Liles, 1979). Aphasic persons retain subpropositional gesturing, such as emotional facial expression (Buck and Duffy, 1980) and vocal gestures to convey humor (Gardner et al., 1975). A dissociation between propositional and subpropositional gesture occurs with aphasia (Duffy and Buck, 1979), similar to the dissociation of these two levels of language function in aphasia. Duffy, Duffy, and Mercaitis (1984) were convinced that a pantomime expression deficit in aphasic persons is ". . . an essential rather than accidental feature" of aphasia (p. 272).

Pantomime expressive ability is tested in a manner similar to naming behavior. Employing the *PICA*'s 16-point scoring scale, Duffy and Duffy (1981) found that their aphasic subjects averaged 8.3 with a range of 3.0 to 13.0. The normal range of 10.5 to 13.5 indicated that some aphasic persons pantomime normally when presented a picture of an object. Davis, Artes, and Hoops (1979) found that their aphasic subjects scored higher with pantomimic description of objects than with verbal description. While pantomime may be impaired, it can be a more effective means of communication than verbal expression for some patients. On the other hand, the similarity between the reduced scores of normal and aphasic adults indicates that pantomime without context can be an ambiguous form of communication even without a gesture disorder being present.

Still, many aphasic patients are deficient in production of symbolic gestures. Goodglass and Kaplan (1963) claimed that pantomime production deficit is due to limb apraxia. Duffy and Duffy (1981) argued that limb apraxia does not necessarily cause this problem in aphasic persons and that pantomime deficit is more often due to a central conceptual disorder (i.e., asymbolia) that also produces the verbal symbol deficits of aphasia. A purely symbolic disorder of pantomime production is possible if limb apraxia is either not present or cannot account for the pantomime deficit. However, the presence of limb apraxia upon imitation is common with aphasia. Duffy and Duffy's (1981) aphasic subjects had limb apraxia and pantomime deficit, but statistical analysis indicated that these disorders could not be causally related. An aphasic patient simply may have two different movement disorders. Asymbolia has been proposed as an explanation for the pantomime deficit, because of the co-occurrence of receptive and expressive deficits (i.e., a "central" deficit), correlations between severity of pantomime deficit and severity of language deficits, and an association between type of pantomime deficit and type of aphasia.

Pantomime production was studied in one subject with Broca's and one with Wernicke's aphasia (Duffy et al., 1984). This study was carried out with a new information condition created by having the experimenter seated next to the subject who was to communicate the identity of an object to a receiver seated across from the subject. Pictures of objects were kept out of view of the receiver. As in Buck and Duffy's (1980) study, subjects' gestures were scored based on accuracy of the receiver. The receivers were accurate only 55 and 57 per cent of the time for the two subjects. Moreover, the number and rate of limb movements paralleled the verbal fluency of each subject. This result is similar to Cicone's observation of gestures during interviews with Broca's and Wernicke's aphasic subjects (Cicone, Wapner, Foldi, Zurif, and Gardner, 1979). Duffy and coworkers (1984) concluded that these results support the idea that pantomime deficiency is an essential component of aphasia.

Summary and Conclusion. Aphasic persons retain subpropositional gesture that includes gesticulation, natural expressive movements, affective displays, and indicative movements (i.e., manipulation of common objects for natural purposes and in natural situations). Many patients possess limb apraxia as exhibited in imitation of gesture and following instruction to manipulate objects. We are concerned about this deficit, not because it is a threat to communicative ability by itself, but because it may interfere with steps to train the propositional use of symbolic gesture.

Training in the use of pantomime may be necessary for some patients, because they have difficulty "naming" objects with pantomimic symbols, a disorder that appears to be a reflection of asymbolia. The problem with symbolic gestures was thought to result from a seepage of limb apraxia into the spontaneous production of emblems and pantomimes. Duffy and

Duffy (1981) concluded that limb apraxia "may be a contributing factor in some cases" (p. 82), but most cases of deficient symbolic gesture are probably a result of cognitive disturbances that also produce aphasia.

Not all persons with aphasia are impaired in pantomime recognition and expression. While group averages have been reduced relative to normal controls, many patients demonstrate normal capabilities in the symbolic use of gesture. Furthermore, spontaneous pantomime can be inherently vague, so that some reduced scores with respect to a scoring criterion of perfection do not necessarily mean that a gesture disorder is present. Therefore, asymbolia may not be the basis for aphasia in all cases. To paraphrase Duffy and coworkers (1984), limb apraxia is a nonessential and accidental occurrence with aphasia, while asymbolic deficit is not an accidental feature but also is not an essential feature of aphasia. A patient may have limb apraxia, asymbolia for gesture, both, or neither.

CONVERSATION

Because conversation consists of an interaction structure that differs from traditional clinical observation, clinicians have been interested in determining whether language skills of aphasic clients are different in conversation. The *Functional Communication Profile*, for example, was developed to assess language comprehension and production as it occurs in 'functional'' context, as opposed to the "clinical" contexts of more standard assessment paradigms (Taylor, 1965). Conversation has been viewed as the predominant behavioral format in which naturalistic use of language occurs, as opposed to less frequent formats such as giving a speech, listening to a speech, reading, and writing. While word retrieval skill during conversation (vs. picture naming) is of interest, our primary concern in this chapter is with behaviors that are inherent to conversation as outlined in Chapter 1. The three contexts are utilized within this interactional structure.

Housekeeping Moves and Turn-Taking

While traditional clinical interactions involve the aphasic patient in either repetitive listening or repetitive speaking, conversation consists of both roles being performed in alternation. In a conversation, the aphasic participant would be switching back and forth between these two roles. Questions about aphasia pertain to whether patients initiate speaking turns, whether they engage in appropriate switching behavior, and whether typical housekeeping moves (e.g., gesticulation) are employed in maintaining and switching these roles. As "caricatures" of two types of aphasia, Jaffe (1978) proposed that Broca's aphasia is an impairment of the speaking role, leaving the patient "locked in" the listening role. Even right hemiplegia contributes to this conversational impairment, because usual right-handed gesticulations could not be performed. Wernicke's aphasia, on the other hand, would be a disruption of the listening role, leaving the patient locked in the speaking role. The self-monitoring problem of these patients makes them "charming conversationalists" who do not make any sense. These patients indeed somtimes tend to be talking when they should be listening.

Schienberg and Holland (1980) investigated the question of whether persons with Wernicke's aphasia have difficulty with turn-taking. They applied turn-taking analysis (e.g., Sacks et al., 1974) to the description of two such patients conversing with each other. The investigators concluded that these subjects were not impaired in turn-taking, as evidenced, for example, by minimal overlapping of turns and by use of various techniques for choosing who would be the next speaker. Therefore, there is little support in this study for Jaffe's proposals as they might affect turn-taking per se, even though different aphasias will present disruptions within a listening or speaking turn. Schienberg and Holland concluded that aphasia does not involve impairment of turn-taking.

Substantive Moves

Communication obstacles are common when one participant has aphasia. First, as listeners, aphasic persons may have difficulty understanding the speaker's meaning, or sometimes normal speakers produce awkward forms that are especially difficult for the aphasic person to comprehend. However, one study demonstrated that patients are able to use contingent queries when speaker attempts are ambiguous (Apel, Newhoff, and Browning-Hall, 1982). In a speaking turn, the patient often has difficulty getting his or her idea across on the first attempt. The normal listener often deals with the patient's unsuitable message by making a guess as to what the message was. As indicated in Chapter 1, Lubinski and coworkers (1980) referred to these events as *hint-and-guess* sequences in which a patient's speaking attempt is characterized as a "hint." The clinician or spouse makes a guess, and then the patient responds to the guess.

The following provides some examples of hint-and-guess outcomes as they were defined in the previous chapter:

                                               Hint: I bate the brunch.
                                               Guess: You *ate* the brunch?
    Resolution   Reply: Yes, I did.
                                               Hint: I ate the round one.

	Guess: The cookie?
Breakdown	Reply: No. Not that.
	Guess: The egg.
Revision	Hint: No. Round one and hole in it.
	Guess: Doughnut!
Repair	Reply: Yes. Poe. . . no. . . dough. . . nut.

A few aphasic subjects have demonstrated an ability to revise or repair most turns within the limits of their language disorder (Lubinski et al., 1980). Our example indicates that revision and repair are so similar that these terms are often used synonymously for any adjustment made in response to a breakdown. In another study, the ability to revise was assessed by contriving breakdowns, as in an experimenter's use of a contingent query (e.g., "What did you say?") in response to aphasic subjects' conversational speaking attempts (Newhoff, Tonkovich, Schwartz, and Burgess, 1982). Newhoff found that subjects attempted to revise in response to most queries. Therefore, it appears that aphasic persons retain resolving and revising/repairing substantive moves.

CONVEYING GIVEN AND NEW INFORMATION

Assessments of aphasic language behavior have included attempts to create a new information condition, in which the situation is structured so that the aphasic patient should assume that the evaluator-listener does not know what the patient is about to convey (e.g., DeRenzi and Ferrari, 1978). Three of these were mentioned in this chapter (Buck and Duffy, 1980; Duffy et al., 1984; Kimbarow and Brookshire, 1983). The earlier discussion of agrammatism and referential coherence indicated that persons with Broca's aphasia maintain a sense for what a listener already knows, even from immediately preceding linguistic context (i.e., Gleason et al., 1975). In Kimbarow and Brookshire's study, the experimenters listened to descriptions of videotaped vignettes that aphasic subjects had observed without the experimenters present. Across several trials with the same person in one-person vignettes, subjects decreased their pronoun reference. This progressive decrease indicated that they were sensitive to information becoming known to the listener, as were the normal adults in Krauss and Weinheimer's study (see Chapter 1).

Kimbarow and Brookshire's (1983) data indicate that mildly to moderately impaired aphasic persons of any variety adhere to the given and new contract by taking the point of view of the listener as a conversation might progress. This aspect of conversation has not been studied often with aphasic subjects, and, as indicated elsewhere in this chapter, linguistic and paralinguistic devices that differentiate given and new information may form the basis of future research.

SPEAKER MEANING

In a conversation, a speaker's intended meaning is not necessarily the literal meaning of an utterance. For a listener to receive a speaker's meaning, the listener often must relate the utterance to external and internal contexts, as explained in Chapter 1. In traditional clinical practice with aphasic adults, this feature of natural communication has neither been assessed nor exercised in treatment. Usually aphasic patients are observed with respect to literal meaning. The most basic difference between speaker meaning and sentence meaning occurs when the form of a sentence does not correspond to a speaker's intention in the form of a speech act.

Studies of aphasia have shown that there is a dissociation between speech acts and sentence production, in which sentence production is impaired but ability to express intentions, including requests, remains intact (Guilford and O'Conner, 1982; Prinz, 1980). In spite of their ability to convey varied intentions, aphasic persons seem to be constrained in their use of speech acts in the clinic, even in conversations with clinicians (Kimbarow, 1982; Wilcox and Davis, 1977). Frequent questioning and stimulating by clinicians promotes frequent asserting by patients, a clinical interaction style that Kimbarow called "therapizing." In this section, we shall explore the aphasic person's ability to comprehend a speaker's intended meaning.

Indirect Requests

The dissociation between speaker meaning and sentence adequacy has also been seen in receptive function, as aphasic persons are able to comprehend indirect requests conveyed in natural contexts. Wilcox, Davis, and Leonard (1978) presented video recordings of brief communicative interactions between two adults to a mixed group of aphasic subjects. Each vignette contained linguistic and contextual information (e.g., A person is standing in front of a door with an armload of books. Another person walks by, and the person with the books asks, "Can you open the door?"). The listener in each episode responded appropriately (i.e., an action) or literally (i.e., "Yes") to a variety of indirect request forms (e.g., "Should you. . . ?", "Will you. . . ?"). Aphasic subjects usually preferred the nonliteral, action response to an indirect request. Furthermore, subjects performed much better than their scores on standard tests of literal comprehension might have predicted.

Hirst, LeDoux, and Stein (1984) sharpened the focus of Wilcox's research paradigm by examining only subjects with Broca's aphasia and their ability to comprehend only the conventional "Can you. . . ?" form of indirect request. The investigators were particularly interested in whether aphasic persons' comprehension of indirect requests depends on an ability to comprehend the literal meaning of the requests. This dependence comprises part of the three-stage model of nonliteral interpretation mentioned in Chapter 1. Two basic experimental conditions were created in which context determined whether a "Can you. . . ?" form should be interpreted literally as a question or nonliterally as an indirect request. Results showed that aphasic subjects' judgments about indirect requests were comparable to normal controls, indicative of an ability to understand these intentions as found by Wilcox and coworkers (1978). However, the aphasic subjects had difficulty judging when a "Yes" was appropriate in the question condition. Hirst concluded that comprehension of literal meaning is not a necessary ingredient in the comprehension of conventional indirect requests. This study also revealed another version of the dissociation between literal and nonliteral comprehension in aphasia.

Metaphor

Metaphor is another vehicle for assessing a person's sensitivity to language-context interactions. Holland (1980) acknowledged this with her use of two "stored" metaphors (i.e., idioms) in her test *Communicative Abilities in Daily Living*. Metaphor is a vehicle for tapping into several pragmatic dimensions of language behavior: (a) actual meaning of an utterance in conversation is always in the mind of the user and not always literally in sentence meaning; (b) prior knowledge of the world is an important ingredient in the comprehension process, and metaphor induces processes similar to those involved in comprehending implausible utterances; (c) creative or "fresh" metaphors appear initially to break the cooperation maxim of truthfulness, but through conversational implicature a listener finds truth by relating the utterance to internal and external contexts.

Aphasic individuals appear to be sensitive to nonliteral meanings of metaphor, as they are with indirect requests. Stachowiak used linguistic and extralinguistic contexts in a study involving stored metaphor or idiom (Stachowiak, Huber, Poeck, and Kerschensteiner, 1977). A preceding paragraph provided one context, and pictures in response choices provided the other. Each paragraph (e.g., about a card game) was read to aphasic subjects, and the fourth statement was an idiom such as "The others strip him right down to his shirt." These subjects were as effective as normal controls in selecting a picture representing nonliteral interpretation.

Winner and Gardner (1977) studied comprehension of two types of metaphor, both of which might be mixtures of the fresh and dead variety defined in Chapter 1. Psychological-physical metaphors consist of an adjective drawn from the physical world to express a psychological state (e.g., "He has a heavy heart"). Cross-sensory metaphors involve an adjective related to one sensory modality in order to modify and element from a different sensory domain (e.g., "The music was colorful"). Subjects were presented such statements along with a choice of four pictures, one depicting the metaphoric interpretation, another depicting the literal interpretation, and two others depicting elements of each metaphor. Normal controls chose the metaphoric interpretation 73 per cent of the time. Aphasic subjects chose the metaphoric picture (58 per cent) more often than did the right hemisphere damaged subjects (43 per cent). Errors by aphasic subjects tended to consist of other foils, and they tended to reject the literal foils as being absurd. On the other hand, the right hemisphere damaged subjects often selected literal meaning as their erroneous choice, even though it was sometimes ridiculous.

Brain damaged adults have been studied primarily with respect to the comprehension of dead or stored metaphors (i.e., idioms). As discussed in Chapter 1, these metaphors are very common, and their literal meaning is often implausible or impossible. Yet, with aphasic subjects, implausible statements have been shown to be more difficult to comprehend than plausible statements. The ease of comprehending idioms may be related to their frequent use and to the implausiblity of the literal option. Ability to integrate contextual information may be put to a greater test with the study of context-dependent metaphors, or statements that make sense literally but are used nonliterally in a particular context.

SUMMARY AND CONCLUSION

With respect to the domain of pragmatics, aphasic adults demonstrate many communicative abilities and a few deficits that may interfere with communication. These strengths and weaknesses have been observed in research designed to examine the use of linguistic, paralinguistic, and extralinguistic contexts, as well as in examinations of the effects of these contexts on specific language behaviors. Also, aphasic individuals have been observed in the most common natural paradigm of linguistic performance, namely, conversation. Most aphasic persons appear to be able to employ the rules of behavior that are inherent to conversation. However, with respect to the processing of particular components of context, mild deficits may be found in many cases, and worrisome impairments may be seen in cases of Wernicke's and global aphasia (i.e., in patients with serious auditory language comprehension deficit).

Therefore, it would be worthwhile to assess pragmatic communicative capacities in aphasic clients not only so that we know what our patients can do but also that we might identify contextual impairments that *may* need our attention in treatment.

Chapter 3

Clinical Assessment of Communicative Behavior

In this chapter we intend to present guidelines and suggestions and review current practices relative to the assessment of communicative behavior from a pragmatic perspective. The pragmatic assessment of aphasia has a brief history. In fact, its development is still unfolding, and this chapter represents a status report rather than a final solution. An explicit stimulant to the pragmatic assessment of aphasic communicative behavior was provided by Holland (1975) when she urged clinical aphasiologists to focus more on communicative adequacy and less on linguistic impairments. Holland's suggestion was based upon her observation of the fact that many aphasic patients are able to communicate meaning to a listener in spite of rather severe linguistic limitations. Since Holland's original observations and subsequent suggestions, various clinical aphasiologists and researchers have attempted to examine aspects of aphasic persons' communicative function independent of their linguistic impairments. The result of such examinations has been a growing body of information applicable to the pragmatic assessment of adult aphasia.

We shall discuss two applications of pragmatics to the assessment of aphasic patients' communicative abilities. One involves identification and description of various pragmatic abilities (e.g., use of contextual cues, comprehension of indirect meaning, and conversational regulatory strategies such as housekeeping moves). However, as was seen in Chapter 2, many of these abilities are relatively unimpaired in the face of aphasia. Hence, the second and potentially most useful application of pragmatics is more in line with Holland's recommendations and focuses upon the ways in which aphasic persons utilize their pragmatic abilities to engage in effective communicative interactions.

In Chapter 2, as we were reviewing research in pragmatics, we discussed numerous techniques and procedures that were designed to elicit or examine various pragmatic abilities and their effects upon communicative effectiveness. With some modifications, many of these procedures may ultimately prove useful for purposes of clinical assessment. We believe that the real test of clinical assessment is the degree to which a particular procedure can (a) objectively delineate the parameters to be assessed, (b) be efficiently and reliably administered, and (c) yield information pertinent to the formulation of treatment plans and procedures.

CHALLENGES OF PRAGMATIC ASSESSMENT

A variety of challenges face the creation and application of pragmatically based clinical assessments as attempts are made to meet the criteria of clinical usefulness. An initial challenge that is very practical in nature pertains to the selection of appropriate assessment content. There is a strong need for guidelines relative to assessment content. As is apparent from Chapter 1, pragmatics is a vast area. The task of identifying relevant and important parameters for assessment content surely is overwhelming. This selection process is further complicated by the dual focus of a clinical pragmatic assessment: (a) the need to identify a given patient's specific pragmatic strengths and weaknesses and (b) determining the ways in which these strengths and weaknesses contribute to overall communicative effectiveness. Obviously, not all pragmatic parameters comprise appropriate assessment content for all aphasic persons. Even if such a "complete" assessment were appropriate, it could take months. In meeting the challenge of assessment content it will be necessary to generate guidelines that can be used in order to select appropriate assessment content for a given patient.

A second challenge facing pragmatic assessments concerns the objective delineation of pragmatic parameters. A first step toward meeting the requirement of objectivity involves construction of operational definitions of the various pragmatic parameters that capture the essence of natural communication yet can still be observed in a clinical setting. This sort of operational specification is difficult because (a) the area of pragmatics itself is ever changing and (b) many variables often operate in combination with the combinatory effects frequently being subject to a variety of influences. The broad and ever growing body of pragmatic variables in and of itself creates a cumbersome situation for constructing appropriate and accurate definitions. When this is coupled with the need to consider various combinations of pragmatic behavior, the task becomes even more formidable.

To illustrate some of the difficulties with operational definitions let us consider formulation of a definition for *referential coherence*. We know from Chapter 1 that one way such coherence is accomplished in normal speakers is through the use of linguistic devices such as definite articles, indefinite articles, pronouns, and causal relationships. Thus a working definition of referential coherence might be:

> The use of an indefinite article for the first mention, and the use of definite articles for second mention. For pronouns, a noun is used for first mention and then a pronoun may only be used for second mention. In the case of causal relations, a verb is used that clearly establishes a link between propositions.

Now, let us attempt to apply this definition to the analysis of aphasic communicative behavior. First, we know that most aphasic patients have word retrieval difficulties, thereby increasing the probability of problems in producing a specific verb to establish a causal link. We also know from Chapter 2 that many aphasic persons omit articles (Gleason et al., 1975) and overuse pronouns (Kimbarow and Brookshire, 1983). Even though the aphasic subjects in both of these investigations omitted these linguistic coherence devices, it was reported that they were careful to ensure that their listeners could identify the referents. If we were to evaluate aphasic patients' coherence abilities on the basis of our working definition, then they would probably be judged as having difficulty with referential coherence. Of course, this sort of misjudgment could be avoided by creating a broader definition of referential coherence as in:

> The speaker somehow ensures that the listener can identify the appropriate referents.

Given the fact that we expect aphasic patients to exhibit difficulty with retrieval of specific linguistic devices, this second definition may be regarded as more appropriate when evaluating aphasic communication. However, the problem with this definition is the fact that it places a large reliance on listener sophistication and, potentially, listener familiarity. Some listeners may be able to identify referents whereas others, given the same situation and information, may not. Although listener sophistication and familiarity is a communicative reality capable of affecting many aphasic persons' communicative effectiveness, it is an undesirable confound when attempting to operationally define a particular communicative skill.

The problems in operationally defining pragmatic variables are by no means limited to referential coherence. Most pragmatic behavior is a result of a combination of influences that vary as a function of different contexts, and differing listeners are often one influential contextual factor. We could, of course, attempt to conceptualize and define variables that are independent of contexts and listeners, and upon first thought, this sort of approach might seem to be a reasonable solution to the problem of creating widely applicable operational definitions. However, by definition, pragmatics is a study of the use of language in context; and context, as we know is rarely a constant variable. What may be appropriate at one time and in one setting may not necessarily be appropriate in another. What may be communicatively effective in an interaction with one listener may not necessarily be effective with another. Thus attempts to define behavior that do not consider contextual variables would result in a set of definitions that are not pragmatic in nature.

Although we have presented a number of difficulties inherent in the process of defining pragmatic behavior, we do not mean to suggest that operational definitions are impossible to create. Various clinicians, ourselves included (see Chapter 1), have attempted to define aspects of pragmatic behavior (e.g., Gurland et al., 1982; Holland, 1980, 1982; Prutting and Kirchner, 1983). The definitions resulting from such exemplary attempts have, for the most part, acknowledged the interaction of context and behavior. The important factor, for clinical assessment, is to use or create definitions of pragmatic behavior that are sensitive to contextual effects while also retaining enough clarity to be reliably applied across a variety of observers.

A third challenge facing pragmatic assessment is the need to preserve a degree of naturalness in a clinical, that is, unnatural communicative setting. If we wish to observe aspects of natural communicative behavior, then we need to create a setting that is conducive to the elicitation of that behavior. The problem facing the preservation of naturalness is in many ways similar to a problem facing the construction of appropriate operational definitions, that is, the combinatory effect of pragmatic behavior. In natural communicative interactions pragmatic behavior occurs as a combinatory effect whereby persons make use of linguistic, paralinguistic, and extralinguistic parameters. In many cases it may be difficult to ensure the availability of natural contextual variables in a contrived setting. The ability to create a more natural setting will be largely facilitated by adequate operational definitions of the behavior to be assessed. If a particular parameter is clearly defined, then a clinical aphasiologist will know the situation that must be created in order to observe occurrence of the target behavior.

The final challenge of pragmatic assessments concerns the relationship between assessment and treatment. This challenge is by no means unique to pragmatics. The gap between assessment and treatment has been of concern to speech-language pathologists for years. Ideally, a clinically useful assessment should generate information that evolves into a treatment plan. In the case of pragmatic assessments this information should include (a) an inventory of successful and unsuccessful communicative strategies, (b) an analysis of fluctuation in communicative behavior as a function of contextual variables, and (c) specific procedures that may be used to elicit from or focus an aphasic patient upon successful communicative strategies.

Overall, pragmatic appraisals face a variety of challenges in an attempt to achieve psychometric elegance while also preserving naturalness and clinical utility. Foldi and colleagues (1983) considered the psychometric problem in terms of "a kind of linguistic indeterminancy principle: The challenge has been to observe the phenomenon of naturalistic communication without destroying it in the process" (p. 53). As clinical aphasiologists, we would add our own comments to those of Foldi and coworkers: The challenge is not only to observe the natural phenomenon but to gain an understanding of the process such that effective remediation can be implemented. Thus, the challenges of pragmatic assessment, for the clinical aphasiologist, primarily concern (a) achieving reliability, which is met by creating conditions that can be administered consistently, (b) the creation of operational definitions that capture true pragmatic ability while also yielding unambiguous and consistent scoring techniques, (c) the specification of important assessment content, and (d) the specification of information that can easily translate into a treatment plan.

CONTENT OF PRAGMATIC ASSESSMENTS

Our initial discussion of pragmatic assessments will focus upon the challenge presented with respect to content selection. That is, precisely "what" should be the focus of a pragmatic assessment? As we have previously acknowledged, pragmatics is an extremely broad area and the clinical problem is to pare it down in such a way that meaningful information can be gained about a patient's communicative abilities. The "whats" of pragmatic assessment have been approached from various viewpoints. Some have attempted to gain an overall picture of communicative functioning whereas others have focused upon identification of specific communicative strategies. Most of the studies reported in Chapter 2 had this latter focus, while most aphasiologists concerned with assessment have had the former focus. Both orientations are clinically important. It is as important to understand the entire process as it is to analyze the component parts and their relative contribution to the global communicative process. The difficulty comes in an attempt to determine the relative contribution of a given parameter to the overall process. This difficulty is further compounded in the face of aphasia.

Strategies that are intact and effective for some patients may not necessarily be intact *and* effective for others. Given this rather individualized nature of pragmatics, particularly in aphasia, the selection of appropriate assessment content can become a rather frustrating task.

Fortunately, a variety of research has been conducted in the area of aphasia and pragmatics. Many of these studies, which were discussed in Chapter 2, have yielded information that is applicable for the formulation of appropriate assessment content. The task is to integrate the information in such a way that a global set of guidelines is created. Our attempt at such an integration is displayed in Table 3-1. The table represents an organization and summary of the research that was presented in Chapter 2. This table can be viewed as an initial set of guidelines that provide the clinical aphasiologist with information relative to expected pragmatic strengths and limitations and thereby generally specify aspects of assessment content. The next step is the process of examining the degree to which an expected strength or limitation either contributes to or hinders effective communicative interactions.

In addition to the content orientation that would result from application of the guidelines in Table 3-1, there is another aspect of communicative behavior in aphasic persons that warrants consideration for assessment content, and this aspect may function somewhat independently of the various contextual influences. That is, many aphasic patients may produce abnormal, but nonetheless communicatively effective, behavior. This type of behavior is often developed by aphasic patients as a means of compensating for their linguistic impairments and has frequently been referred to as *compensatory communicative behavior.* Although such behavior may not necessarily be pragmatically based, it is often pragmatically useful, and assessments should be structured so as to identify the use or degree of effectiveness of such compensatory behavior.

The initial "whats" of pragmatic assessment can be conceptualized in two ways. One includes a content focus upon pragmatic strengths and limitations, and the second includes a focus upon behavior that may have developed as a means of compensating for linguistic impairment. In order to analyze the effects of each of the parameters a clinical aphasiologist will need to examine verbal as well as nonverbal behavior.

Verbal Behavior: Contextual Influences

Verbal expression as well as comprehension is often subject to linguistic, paralinguistic, and extralinguistic influences. Hence, each of these contextual variables may merit consideration for the content of pragmatic assessments. Table 3-1 provides general guidelines relative to each of these contextual parameters. The assessment process therefore

Table 3–1. Summary of Pragmatic Abilities in Aphasia

Linguistic Contextual Strengths
  Knowledge and use of discourse macrostructures
  Ability to maintain referential coherence in spite of article
    omissions and overuse of pronouns
  Semantic plausibility facilitates comprehension

Parlinguistic Contextual Strength
  Comprehension and use of prosody expressing emotion
  Production of prosody in fluent aphasias
  Exaggerated stress facilitates comprehension of lexical items

Extralinguistic Contextual Strengths
  Recognition of auditory and other nonverbal components of a setting
  Conceptual knowledge pertaining to topics of conversation
  Appropriate emotional states
  Knowledge and recognition of roles of conversational participants
  Some movement including facial expression (usually unilateral in nonfluent aphasias
    and bilateral in fluent aphasias)
  Use of pointing to supplement verbal expression

Conversational Strengths: Interaction of Contexts
  Appropriate use of turn-taking rules for conversation, including relatedness, repairs,
    provision of feedback (i.e., contingent queries), and minimal overlap.
  Sensitivity to the conversational cooperative principle
  Sensitivity to given and new information distinctions (i.e., point of view of a listener)
  Comprehension of speaker intentions and meaning (e.g., nonliteral interpretation of
    conventional indirect requests and metaphor)

Contextual and Conversational Limitations
  Occasional failure to comprehend pronoun coreference
  Agrammatic omission of articles to distinguish given and new information
  Incoherent semantic shifts in jargon of Wernicke's aphasia
  Moderate difficulty comprehending emotional prosody in severe aphasia
  Impaired comprehension of semantic and syntactic uses of prosody
  Some auditory agnosia for environmental sounds in patients with severe language
    comprehension deficits
  Possible disorganization of conceptual knowledge in severe aphasia
  Difficulty in using symbolic movement patterns

---

becomes one of determining the degree to which an expected strength or limitation may affect communicative effectiveness. For example, an expected strength for most aphasic patients is the ability to use extralinguistic context (e.g., pointing) in order to supplement verbal information. In the assessment process it would be important to examine (a) the degree to which a patient might rely on this strategy and (b) the degree to which a patient experiences success with this strategy.

Another example relative to the application of the guidelines pertains to turn-taking abilities. Most aphasic patients retain knowledge relative to turn-taking. One aspect of turn-taking is the ability to repair a message when a listener indicates a lack of comprehension. When a patient is confronted with negative listener feedback it would be important to note (a) strategies they may use to repair a message and (b) the successfulness of particular repair strategies.

As an additional example, let us consider an expected limitation in many aphasic patients: the omission of articles to distinguish given and new information. It would be important to note the degree to which this limitation actually interferes with the ability to convey given and new distinctions. If the interference is minimal (i.e., given and new distinctions are made in spite of article omission), then it becomes important to note the ways in which a patient manages to maintain given and new distinctions for a listener.

As a final example, we shall consider the effects of paralinguistic information on linguistic comprehension. Many aphasic patients have demonstrated difficulties in utilizing prosody as a cue for the comprehension of propositional intents such as declaratives and interrogatives (Green and Boller, 1974; Heilman et al., 1984). Additionally, patients with Broca's aphasia were found to have difficulty in using stress to comprehend otherwise ambiguous sentences such as "They are *fighting* dogs" versus "They are fighting *dogs*" (Baum et al., 1982). Since these sorts of paralinguistic cues are frequently critical to conversational comprehension (see Chapter 1) it would be important to determine the degree to which this limitation may result in communicative difficulties as well as any potential compensatory mechanisms a patient may have developed. On the more positive side, Pashek and Brookshire (1982) have found that exaggerated stress on crucial lexical items facilitates paragraph comprehension in aphasia. Although in the normal conversation process exaggerated stress is used to highlight new information, it would still be important to determine the degree to which this paralinguistic strength might offset or minimize the noted paralinguistic limitations.

The guidelines in Table 3-1 specify the major contextual influences on communicative behavior and as such constitute *potentially* appropriate content for pragmatic assessments. The list in Table 3-1 is by no means exhaustive, it is merely a beginning. The guidelines were designed to be generally applicable to aphasic patients; however, not all patients will demonstrate the expected strengths, nor will all patients demonstrate the expected limitations.

Compensatory Verbal Behavior

We shall now focus upon that behavior we have described as pragmatic in function but not necessarily a component of the pragmatic rules of conversation. Many aphasic patients produce verbal behavior that is abnormal yet communicatively effective. These types of compensatory behavior are frequently developed by patients in response to their linguistic impairments; therefore they are not typically influenced by contextual variables. Gleason and coworkers (1975) identified strategies used by patients with Broca's aphasia as a means of compensating for their syntactic deficits. The strategies included (a) a *search for a stressed opening word,* such as a vocative in "Cousin, sit down"; (b) the use of *adverbs* to express future tense, as in "He work again next week" or to express the comparative, as in "She is tall enough"; and (c) *concatenated phrases,* whereby constituents are placed in a series instead of being embedded as in "a large house, a white house."

Self-correction is another compensatory ability that some aphasic persons possess and others develop during their recovery. This strategy depends upon an individual's ability to recognize his or her own errors, and it is this self-recognition that differentiates self-corrections from the conversational repairs that were previously discussed as an aspect of turn-taking. Marshall and Tompkins (1981, 1982) identified three categories of unassisted self-correction through their observations of aphasic subjects' communicative behavior during short-answer and single-word tasks. The categories included cued correction, effortful correction, and immediate correction. *Cued corrections* occurred when a patient produced a related response, or responses prior to the target response, as in "Truck, no, uh car, yes *car.*" *Effortful corrections* occurred when a patient produced a series of partial responses prior to the target responses, as in "tair, no, uh t. . . , ch. . . , un chair, yes *chair.*" Immediate corrections were those in which a patient was able to easily correct a misproduction, as in "uck, *truck.*"

Marshall (1976) as well as Farmer (1977) examined the use and success of various word retrieval strategies in a variety of aphasic patients. Marshall identified five strategies including (a) *delay,* taking or requesting time to retrieve a word; (b) *semantic paraphasia,* such as "This is my rocking chair . . ." (for wheelchair); (c) *phonetic association,* which included phonemic paraphasias, such as "Last night we had trod, trat, trot (trout) for dinner"; (d) *circumlocution,* in which a description of a target word is provided, as in "It's that place where you go to take a bath"; and (e) *generalization,* which is the production of indefinite words instead of content words, as in "It the one there, it a one." Farmer used categories similar to those identified by Marshall. The results of both investigations indicated that the delay strategy was the most effective with respect to retrieval of an intended word, and Farmer found this to be the most frequently employed strategy. However, Marshall found semantic paraphasias to be the most frequent strategy and reported that delays were relatively rare.

These descriptions of some types of compensatory behavior can provide a general orientation relative to potential assessment content. Although aphasic patients may demonstrate many commonalities in their compensatory mechanisms, they may also demonstrate a large degree of uniqueness. Also, some behavior may be clearly compensatory in nature and not particularly effective. Assessments should be constructed such that compensatory behavior can be identified and evaluated relative to its contribution to communicative effectiveness.

Nonverbal Behavior

In addition to verbal behavior, pragmatic assessments should include an analysis of nonverbal behavior. In many aphasic patients the majority of their communicative adaptations may be expressed in the nonverbal mode. Analysis of nonverbal behavior should focus upon intentional as well as unintentional components. Intentional components can be defined as behavior that is produced by the person in order to convey some information to a listener. Unintentional behavior may have communicative value to a listener but it is not intentionally produced for purposes of communication. The content of nonverbal analyses should be the same as that which was described for verbal analyses. The guidelines listed in Table 3–1 should be applied in order to determine effects of pragmatic strengths and limitations on nonverbal behavior. Further, nonverbal behavior should be examined in order to identify potential compensatory strategies.

Unfortunately, nonverbal behavior is a much broader realm than verbal behavior. Initially it is crucial to have an idea as to ways in which nonverbal behavior might be categorized (other than intentional versus unintentional). Our attempt to categorize aspects of nonverbal behavior is displayed in Table 3–2. The table includes a summary of most gestures studied in people with aphasia but certainly does not include all possible gestures. Most of the gestures we have identified are considered to be communicative, either at a propositional (i.e., intentional) or subpropositional (i.e., unintentional) level. Our classification often represents ends of continuums rather than mutually exclusive entities. Propositionality, for example, is a continuum; and iconicity is a continuum. Our classification system is not intended to represent resolved issues of terminology. For example, some may consider pantomime to be nonsymbolic. Our placement of categories is primarily based upon clinical

Table 3-2. Categories of Nonverbal Behavior

Symbolic Gestures
  Iconic (representative of referent)
    Pantomime (directly representational; often transitive)
    Natural gestures used propositionally
    Other (e.g., numbers)
  Arbitrary
    Emblems (conventional, often intransitive)
    Formal symbolic codes (e.g., American Sign Language)
    Writing in the air

Signals
  Gesticulations (conversational regulators accompanying speech)
  Natural expressive gestures (e.g., frowning when puzzled)
  Affective displays (e.g., facial expressions)
  Indicative movements (e.g., demonstrating object use with object present)

precedent and is our attempt to lend some structure to the content of pragmatic analysis.

Upon examining the table it can be seen that our initial category includes symbolic gestures. *Symbolic gestures* are referential in that they represent objects, events, or more abstract concepts. Their use can be described as being intentional. Most symbolic gestures are normally used as substitutes for speech rather than augmentations or supplements. *Iconic* gestures capture the nature of a referent, and they may vary in their degree of iconicity, with some gestures being more representational than others (Harrison, 1974). They include *pantomime*, such as illustrating the use of an object without the object being present. Many pantomimes are considered to be "transitive," because they are displays of an action upon an imagined object; however, they are often used by aphasic patients as a means of simply referring to that object. Pantomime has also been referred to as "representational gesture" (Helm-Estabrooks, Fitzpatrick, and Barresi, 1982). A second type of iconic gesture consists of *natural signal behavior,* such as rubbing one's eyes or scratching one's head, when they are used intentionally to convey sadness or confusion, respectively. A third form of iconic gesture includes the use of one's fingers to express a number.

Arbitrary symbolic gestures bear no physical resemblance to their referents, and some authors consider arbitrariness to be a criterion for a gesture to be symbolic (e.g., Peterson and Kirshner, 1981). The most frequently cited arbitrary gesture system is American Sign Language. Writing in the air is also included in the arbitrary symbol category. Although some may regard American Indian Gestural Code (Amer-Ind) as arbitrary, it is generally thought to be a more iconic code. Emblems or "conventional gestures" may be arbitrary or iconic. Emblems include a salute, crossing oneself, and the common "OK" sign (formulating a circle with the thumb and index finger). Arbitrary gestures are among the "intransitive" symbols, when the gesture is not an action upon an object.

Most *signals*, while they convey information, are defined as being unintentional (i.e., "naturally released," subpropositional), nonsymbolic, or nonreferential. They usually accompany speech and function similarly to the paralinguistic trappings of verbal productions when used for emphasis. *Gesticulation,* discussed in Chapter 1, includes head, arm, and hand movements that regulate conversation turn-taking, as in maintaining or relinquishing a turn as a speaker. Another type of signal is the *natural expressive gesture,* which is often an immediate reaction to a situation such as rubbing eyes while slicing an onion or covering ears in the presence of a painful noise (Goodglass and Kaplan, 1963). A third type of signal is *affective display,* reflecting a person's emotional state. Facial expression often appears as such a signal. Just as a natural expressive gesture can be used propositionally, a facial expression of sadness or anger can also be used intentionally, for example, to convey a feeling experienced in the past. In these instances, the affective display becomes an iconic symbol. Finally, *indicative gestures* are object manipulations with the object present (Peterson and Kirshner, 1981). They are included here because they have been elicited frequently as a means of identifying the presence of limb apraxia and also as a means of assessing gestural communicative ability (e.g., Porch, 1981). They are usually elicited upon request (e.g., "Show me what you do with this"). Indicative gestures differ from pantomime in that in pantomime, the object is not present.

We believe that the classification system presented in Table 3–2 will facilitate pragmatic assessments of nonverbal behavior. At the very least it provides some guidelines that can be used to sort the realm of nonverbal behavior in order to identify contextual influences as well as compensatory mechanisms. Although we have specifically defined the various categories, it is important to remember that a given movement pattern (i.e., gesture) may be a symbol or a sign depending upon its intentionality or propositionality.

Summary of Assessment Content

In this section we have discussed a variety of issues concerning the selection and creation of pragmatic assessment content. Based upon the research that has been conducted in aphasia and pragmatics, we have constructed some initial guidelines that may be used for the formulation of assessment content. These guidelines specify general pragmatic strengths and limitations that one may expect to observe in most aphasia patients. We have recommended that these guidelines be applied to the analysis of verbal and nonverbal behavior and have provided a variety of examples concerning the content of such analyses. Additionally, we have suggested an organizational structure for the content of nonverbal analyses through a discussion of a movement (i.e., gestural) classification system. Finally, in addition to assessment content focusing upon the effects of pragmatic behavior, we have identified the need to focus upon potential compensatory behavior that may be pragmatically useful.

PRAGMATIC ASSESSMENT PROCEDURES

We now turn our attention to procedures that have been or may be used in order to conduct pragmatic assessments. Hence, in this section we discuss a variety of procedures and procedural issues relative to pragmatic assessment and, in doing so, demonstrate the various ways in which clinical aphasiologists have approached the challenges of creating operational definitions, preserving naturalness, and generating information applicable to treatment. Many of the procedures we consider were designed to assess various aspects of pragmatic behavior that we identified in our discussions of assessment content. Therefore, our focus in this procedural section is less on content and more on the variety of ways in which pragmatic behavior may be assessed.

Although many of the procedures discussed demonstrate variety as well as creativity, at this point in time we do not believe that any one technique can be viewed as *the* comprehensive pragmatic procedure. Further, given the ever-growing breadth of pragmatics, it seems unlikely that a single comprehensive procedure will be forthcoming in the near future. However, we do believe it is possible, through application of content guidelines and selection of certain procedures, to create a battery of assessment devices capable of yielding a relatively representative profile of a patient's pragmatic communication abilities.

An initial procedural distinction can be made in terms of formal standardized tests and informal testing techniques. Formal tests represent those instruments for which norms are usually available, and reliability as well as validity have been determined. Informal procedures, on the other hand, utilize principles of scientific observation in order to describe behavior. In terms of content focus, standardized tests are generally designed to yield a general picture of communicative abilities, whereas many informal procedures focus upon gaining information relative to more specific communicative strategies.

One of the earliest investigators to relate pragmatics to assessment in terms of a *formal test* was Sarno (1969) with her *Functional Communication Profile* (FCP). Although the term "pragmatics" was not in common use at the time of the test development, the test incorporates many pragmatic principles. Sarno distinguished natural, everyday language use from language elicited in artificial testing situations. Hence the FCP was designed to provide an estimate of a patient's everyday or natural communicative abilities in terms of verbal reception and expression without actually conducting observations in the natural environment. Sarno emphasized that the FCP was not intended to replace tests of specific linguistic abilities (e.g., *Boston Diagnostic Aphasia Examination,* Goodglass and Kaplan, 1972), but rather was intended to be a supplement to linguistic evaluations. A variety of behavior types are rated in the administration of the FCP. These include indicating yes and no, obtaining information from other people, and reading a newspaper. The behavioral rating is accomplished with a 9-point scale that ranges from normal to absent ability. The FCP is relatively subjective in nature and provides no normative data, although acceptable interjudge reliability coefficient scores have been reported (.87).

More recently, Holland (1980) developed a test entitled *Communicative Abilities in Daily Living* (CADL). As Holland pointed out in her test manual, with the exception of the FCP, clinicians most often are expected to generalize findings from tests assessing linguistic competence to overall communicative effectiveness in daily living situations. Questioning the validity of such generalizations, Holland designed the CADL so as to provide a standardized measure of an aphasic person's everyday communicative skills. Like Sarno, Holland emphasized that the CADL was not intended to replace more linguistically oriented tests. Rather, its purpose is to provide information concerning communicative rather than purely linguistic ability.

The CADL, which can be administered in a clinical setting, simulates natural settings and provides real-life communication problems as tasks. For example, several test items are constructed around the theme of keeping an appointment with a physician. In these situations a tester pretends to be a receptionist (with appropriate props), and the patient is required to do such things as communicate the time of his or her appointment, show identification, and obtain a seat in a crowded waiting room. The test is composed of 68 tasks that are scored as "correct," "adequate," or "wrong." The scores are assigned on the basis of a patient's success in communicating a given message.

Both the FCP and the CADL represent an important component of pragmatic assessment. They provide information concerning an aphasic person's overall communicative effectiveness and, as such, assess the global contribution of a patient's pragmatic strengths and limitations to his or her communicative effectiveness. The CADL, to date, represents the most comprehensive formal attempt to assess aphasic communication pragmatically. However, neither test is designed to identify the individual contributions of specific pragmatic strengths or limitations (e.g., turn-taking ability, use of paralinguistic cues, referential coherence) to overall communicative ability.

The bulk of pragmatically oriented assessments for aphasic adults have been developed as *informal testing procedures*. Although such techniques do not provide normative data, they can yield diverse information relative to a patient's communicative behavior that is directly applicable to treatment planning and implementation. In addition, many informal measures may frequently serve as useful techniques for assessing treatment progress. Our discussion of informal procedures is organized in accordance with the ways in which a behavioral sample may be obtained from an aphasic client. We have created five major categories, including (a) conversational samples, (b) structured tasks, (c) role-playing, (d) questionnaires, and (e) natural observations.

Conversational Samples

Several clinicians have attempted to assess aspects of aphasic discourse behavior by observing face-to-face conversations in a clinical setting (e.g., Davis and Wilcox, 1981; Gurland et al., 1982; Houghton, Pettit, and Towey, 1982; Lubinski et al., 1980; Prutting and Kirchner, 1983; Schienberg and Holland, 1980; Ulatowska, Doyel, Stern, Haynes, and North, 1983; Wilcox and Davis, 1977; Yorkston et al., 1980). In many ways, conversation can be viewed as the best context in which to observe the occurrence and effects of pragmatic behavior. Analyses of face-to-face interactions provide opportunities to assess influences of numerous contextual parameters (e.g., facilitation of linguistic context, familiarity of conversational partners, turn-taking abilities). As in the early development of any clinical methodology, the pioneering efforts have varied, especially with respect to conversational procedures, conversational contexts, and the parameters chosen for description and measurement.

Spontaneous versus Elicited Conversations. Conversations obtained in a clinical setting can be classified as either spontaneous or elicited. *Spontaneous conversation* either involves no instructions or instructions indicating that the participants are to talk about whatever they wish. *Elicited conversation* includes giving the participants a specific topic or pictures to talk about, or an interview format may be employed with the nonaphasic partner asking open-ended questions. Several techniques have been reported for eliciting conversation. One includes a situation in which aphasic clients are asked to communicate information about a picture hidden from the view of a partner (Davis and Wilcox, 1981; Yorkston et al., 1980). Other means of eliciting conversation have included picture descriptions in which the picture is in view of both communicative partners (Spiegel, Jones, and Wepman, 1965) and interviews with open-ended questions (Prinz, Snow, and Wagenaar, 1978). As a specific mechanism for eliciting narrative discourse, Ulatowska and her colleagues have relied upon picture-story sequences and story re-telling tasks (Ulatowska, North, and Macaluso-Haynes, 1981; Ulatowska, Freedman-Stern, Doyel, Macaluso-Haynes, and North, 1983). Procedural discourse has been elicited from aphasic clients by asking them to give instructions as to how to do something, such as changing a light bulb or making a sandwich (Ulatowska, Doyel, Stern, Haynes, and North, 1983).

There are advantages as well as disadvantages in both approaches to sampling conversational discourse. The advantages of an elicited sample compared to a spontaneous sample are that (a) they usually can be accomplished more quickly and (b) they can be structured to enable examination of specific communicative strategies (e.g., narrative discourse with a story re-telling task). However, in order to conduct an effective elicitation task, a clinician needs specific definitions of a behavior to be evaluated. The necessity of such specificity may create a narrower assessment focus than would occur with a spontaneous sample. It is difficult to evaluate overall communicative effectiveness with an elicited task, since it may tend to produce a less natural sample. Further, the nonaphasic partner may frequently resort to a questioning format. Some elicitation tasks (e.g., picture description when a picture is in view of both the aphasic client and his or her partner) are more artificial than others (e.g., interview with open-ended questions). These more artificial tasks typically do not involve a true communication partner. There is no real *need* to communicate information, because it is already known by the participants with a picture in view of both. With these more artificial tasks aspects of face-to-face *interaction*, such as certain conversational regulatory strategies (i.e., housekeeping moves), cannot be effectively evaluated. A final disadvantage of elicited conversational samples concerns the ability to assess aspects of pragmatics with respect to comprehension. Most elicited tasks are designed to focus upon expressive conversational behavior. In fact, it would be difficult to design an elicited task whereby one could assess pragmatic strengths and limitations with respect to comprehension in natural conversations. One could give the patient some information (i.e., produce a discourse) and then ask questions. However, a task such as this could easily resemble a testing situation and seriously hinder the opportunity to observe natural strategies.

The primary advantage of a spontaneous sample is its greater probability of yielding behavior that is representative of a patients' typical communicative abilities in terms of expression as well as comprehension, therefore facilitating an evaluation of a patient's overall communicative effectiveness. Some aspects of face-to-face interaction, such as appropriate use of speech acts and natural comprehension strategies, are easier to observe in a spontaneous sample. However, it should also be noted that any sample obtained in a clinic frequently sacrifices naturalness. Oftentimes, spontaneous conversation arranged in a clinic can seem to be so contrived that it becomes difficult for the participants to think of anything to discuss.

Usually, the goals of an assessment determine the method used to obtain a sample of conversational discourse. If a clinician wants to evaluate overall communicative effectiveness or aspects of behavior more likely to occur in a natural face-to-face interaction, then a spontaneous sample is more appropriate. However, if a clinician has already decided to evaluate specific aspects of pragmatic behavior, then an elicited sample is more efficient. In other words, in many pragmatic assessments there is probably a place for elicited as well as spontaneous sampling techniques.

Sample Length. Lengths reported for conversational samples have varied, the most frequently reported being 15 minutes for spontaneous as well as elicited discourse. Some reports have included samples as long as 60 minutes (e.g., Wilcox and Davis, 1977) and others as short as six minutes (e.g., Lubinski et al., 1980). Although many clinicians have used videotapes and conducted analyses after-the-fact, some clinicians have relied upon on-the-spot analyses. Typically, one sample has been regarded as sufficient for the longer lengths (e.g., Wilcox and Davis, 1977) whereas two or three samples have been obtained for the shorter durations (e.g., Lubinski et al., 1980). We would additionally recommend that the number of samples be increased if videotaping is not feasible. Some investigators, following a tradition established in child language research, have approached length in terms of utterances produced rather than duration (e.g., Florance 1981). Although Florance conducted analyses with samples of 25 utterances, we would recommend, in the tradition established with child language research, that at least 50 and preferably 100 utterances or messages (for less verbal patients) be obtained.

Conversation Analysis Formats. Analyses of conversations have been accomplished in a variety of ways. Some investigators have relied upon subjective rating scales, by which a behavior is rated on a continuum from poor to excellent (e.g., Houghton, et al., 1982). Other investigators have employed more objective scales, rating communicative behavior as a function of completeness of information produced by a patient (e.g., Yorkston et al., 1980) or in relationship to the amount of listener feedback that was required prior to understanding a patient's message (e.g., Davis and Wilcox, 1981). A third way in which pragmatic analyses have also been accomplished includes notations regarding appropriateness versus inappropriateness, or presence or absence of a particular behavior (e.g., Gurland et al., 1982; Prutting and Kirchner, 1983). Finally, many investigators have noted such things as frequency of occurrence, duration, latency, and sequences of specific behavior (e.g., Guilford and O'Connor, 1982; Gurland et al., 1982; Lubinski et al., 1980; Prutting and Kirchner, 1983; Ripich, Terrell, and Spinelli, 1983; Schienberg and Holland, 1980; Wilcox and Davis, 1977).

Observations of Spontaneous Conversations. Numerous types of pragmatic behavior have been observed with informal assessments, and investigators have employed a variety of approaches in attempting to define the behavior being assessed. We shall initially focus our attention upon the types of pragmatic behavior observed in *spontaneous conversations.* Houghton and coworkers (1982) described a procedure called the *Communicative Competence Evaluation Instrument* (CCEI). Observations are made in the form of subjective ratings (no response, poor, fair, average, good, and excellent) for a variety of expressive and receptive communicative behaviors. Receptive behavior includes responses to speech, suprasegmental cues, gross environmental sounds, and the ability to follow gestured and verbal directions. Observations of expressive behavior include demonstration of affect, use of words or gestures to initiate communicative interactions, indication of yes and no, use of verbal and nonverbal listener responses, and indication of acceptance and rejection.

Another approach to observing spontaneous behavior was developed by Prutting and Kirchner (1983). Their procedure takes the form of a checklist of pragmatic behavior and is probably the most comprehensive informal procedure currently available. It is designed for children as well as adults and focuses upon verbal and nonverbal behavior used for expression as well as comprehension. The checklist is organized into three major categories: Utterance acts, propositional acts, and illocutionary or perlocutionary acts. Utterance acts are described as behavior accompanying communicative efforts and include paralinguistic (e.g., prosody, vocal intensity, fluency) and extralinguistic (e.g., facial expressions, gesticulations, posture) variables. Propositional acts refer to actual linguistic productions and include the relationships between words (e.g., word order, given and new distinctions), lexical selections, and stylistic variations. Illocutionary or perlocutionary acts refer to the intentions underlying a communicative effort as well as effects of a communicative effort upon a listener. Behavior in this last category includes turn-taking, topic variables (e.g., appropriate selection, introduction, maintenance, and change), and communicative functions (e.g., request, agree, disagree).

The observation of behavior consists of ratings in the form of "appropriate," "inappropriate," or "no opportunity to observe." In addition to these ratings of appropriateness, Prutting and Kirchner (1983) also generated guidelines for descriptive analyses. These guidelines include the determination of frequency, latency, duration, density, amplitude, and sequences of appropriate and inappropriate behavior.

Gurland and coworkers (1982) used a system originally developed by Wollner and Geller (1982) to observe spontaneous conversations between aphasic clients and their communicative partners. The system provides categories for coding the occurrence of specific behavior produced by the aphasic and nonaphasic communicators. The observational system includes two initial categories: communicative acts and conversational acts. Conversational acts focus primarily upon the *ways* in which a particular topic is initiated, maintained, and terminated. Communicative acts focus more upon the *purposes* of conversations and include descriptions of (a) the ways in which conversation is regulated (e.g., turn-taking, attention getters, polite forms), (b) expression of attitudes, and (c) conveyance of content (e.g., requests, instructions, responses to communications, jokes). In their use of the communication taxonomy, Gurland and coworkers compared observations from their system to CADL scores obtained for two aphasic clients. They concluded that both testing procedures offered indices of clients' communicative abilities and deficits. However, the CADL was found to be more limited in its ability to sample a client's spontaneous conversational skills.

The observational approaches we have considered thus far have been very broad in scope and have focused upon a number of aspects of conversation. Other approaches have been attempted in which a specific pragmatic behavior is assessed through descriptive analysis and frequency counts of spontaneous conversations. These types of behavior have included discourse cohesion, strategies for resolving communicative breakdowns, conversational functions, and turn-taking conventions. Ripich and coworkers (1983) assessed aspects of discourse cohesion at the level of microstructure through determining the presence or absence of ellipses and linguistic devices used to establish referential cohesion. Lubinski and coworkers (1980) analyzed strategies used by aphasic patients and their communicative partners to resolve communicative breakdowns that were created by the aphasic partner. They focused upon attempts that were made by either conversational partner to repair spontaneously occurring breakdowns. Their categories for describing repair strategies included hints, guesses, corrections, and questions produced by the nonaphasic partner, as well as repetitions, corrections, and phonological approximations produced by the aphasic partner.

Guilford and O'Connor (1982) applied Halliday's (1975) distinctions of language function and coded aphasic persons' conversational behavior according to expression of pragmatic functions (use of language to obtain items or to control environmental conditions), mathetic functions (using language to obtain information about or to explore the environment), and informative functions (using language to impart knowledge not shared by a listener). Wilcox and Davis (1977) used Searle's (1969) speech act categories (e.g., agree, assert, disagree, congratulate, warn) to describe aphasic clients' conversational interactions. Schienberg and Holland (1980) described turn-taking behavior in a conversation occurring between two patients with Wernicke's aphasia. They used categories described by Sacks et al. (1974) which focus on such aspects of turn-taking as overlap, turn order, turn size, and turn allocation procedures.

Observations of Elicited Conversation. We shall now turn to the types of pragmatic behavior that have been assesed with *elicited* conversational samples. Davis and Wilcox (1981) and Yorkston and coworkers (1980) assessed aphasic clients' communicative abilities by asking them to talk about pictures that were hidden from the view of a listener. This task, although very contrived, provided the investigators with an opportunity to observe aphasic clients' ability to convey information to a listener effectively. Davis and Wilcox as well as Yorkston and coworkers analyzed their patients performance in this elicited situation by rating their overall communicative effectiveness. Yorkston and coworkers rated communicative effectiveness in terms of the amount (e.g., partial or complete) or type (e.g., relevant or irrelevant) of information a patient was able to convey. Davis and Wilcox rated communicative effectiveness as a function of the amount of listener feedback that was provided before a message was conveyed. A lesser amount of listener feedback (e.g., message was comprehended upon a patient's first transmission) was associated with a more successful message and a larger amount of listener feedback (e.g., one or more contingent queries) was regarded as a less successful communicative attempt. The patient's communicative attempts were assigned a score that was based upon the number of contingent queries a listener produced prior to message comprehension.

Although neither investigation focused upon this issue, the elicited format used by Davis and Wilcox (1981) and Yorkston and coworkers (1980) also provides the opportunity to evaluate the ways in which aphasic patients may differentiate between given versus new information as well as rely on shared versus unshared knowledge. Presumably, the picture hidden from view represents new information. Given information is formulated on the basis of the aphasic person's familiarity with the task as well as the communicative partner. The degree of given information can be varied depending upon whether or not the task has previously been done with the same communicative partner and with the same pictures. Similarly, the degree of new information can be varied by employing unfamiliar pictures and unfamiliar communicative partners.

Other analyses of elicited conversation have examined the content of narrative as well as procedural discourse. Ulatowska, North, and Macaluso-Haynes (1981) and Ulatowska, Freedman-Stern, Doyel, Macaluso-Haynes, and North (1983) analyzed narrative discourse that was obtained with story re-telling, or picture-story tasks. Their analyses included identification of the six steps of discourse macrostructure: (a) an abstract, (b) descriptions of setting involving time, location, and identification of the participants, (c) the order of the action events, (d) an evaluation of what has happened, (e) the result of what has happened, and (f) a moral. Analyses of procedural discourse have typically included identification of three components (a) essential steps, that is, those necessary to perform an action (e.g., "take out the old light bulb"), (b) target steps, that is, those in which one verifies the results of an action (e.g., "turn the switch to see if it works"), and (c) optional steps, that is, those that give more detail or clarify essential steps (e.g., "to remove the bulb you must grab it and turn it counterclockwise").

Structured Tasks. Several clinicians have relied upon structured tasks in order to evaluate specific types of pragmatic behavior. In many ways these tasks resemble elicited conversation. However, in a structured task situation the goal is not to obtain a sample of conversational discourse but rather to manipulate a particular variable and then observe the effects upon communicative behavior. A structured task will not typically be a good starting point for a pragmatic evaluation. Rather, such tasks should be used to further assess aspects of behavior that were deemed "suspect" during a more general evaluation. Many of the research procedures described in Chapter 2 employed structured tasks. Many of these research procedures are not appropriate for clinical assessment as they require equipment and administration time that is unrealistic for a clinical setting. However, other procedures that are relatively quick and simple to administer could easily be incorporated as optional items in an assessment protocol. There are potentially numerous tasks that could be useful for clinical assessment. However, we shall describe only a few in order to illustrate some ways in which a task originally designed for experimental purposes can be used for clinical assessment. We have chosen three tasks that evaluate aphasic clients' use of some important communicative strategies, namely, requesting (either needed items, information, or clarification) and the ability to repair a misunderstood message.

Prinz (1980) described a task designed to elicit *request* behavior. The task includes the creation of situations in which an aphasic person is likely to produce a request. For example, a patient is asked to write his or her name. He or she is given a piece of paper but no pencil. This situation creates a need to request a pencil. Prinz evaluated patients' behavior by noting (a) request attempts and (b) the propositional adequacy of attempted requests.

Apel and coworkers (1982) devised a task in which they created a need for aphasic patients to produce a *contingent query*, that is, request for clarification or additional information. In the task a nonaphasic partner introduces some pictures for discussion with a client. During the course of the discussion the nonaphasic partner makes statements or produces questions containing nonsense words such as "What is the *ruba* doing?" or "That's a nice *kaga*." Apel and coworkers evaluated aphasic clients' responses to these statements by classifying their behavior in one of the following categories:

1. Nonvocal contingent query—any nonverbal indication that further information was desired (e.g., an inquiring look).
2. Vocal contingent query—as in "huh?" or "humm?"
3. Verbal contingent query—the production of some sort of related linguistic behavior (e.g., "Tell you about what?" or "What about the ruba?").
4. Nonrequestive response—the client acted as if the utterance was understood and continued the task.

The structured tasks used by Prinz (1980) and Apel and coworkers (1982) evaluate an important aspect of aphasic communicative behavior, that is, adequacy of request strategies as well as tendencies to produce a request. Although Prinz focused only upon requests for specific items, the task could be redesigned or expanded to include situations in which it is necessary to request information (e.g., the location of a ladies room). Apel and coworkers used nonsense words to create a need to request clarification. This task could easily be made more realistic by eliminating nonsense words and having the partner produce insufficient or inaccurate information. Whether due to a lack of comprehension or insufficient speaker information, aphasic clients may frequently be in situations in which they will need to clearly convey a request for something (e.g., information, objects, clarification). It would therefore seem to be important to evaluate their ability to produce a variety of such requests.

Newhoff and coworkers (1982) analyzed aphasic clients' abilities to repair misunderstood messages with a task that has been widely used in the child language literature (e.g., Gallagher, 1977; Gallagher and Darnton, 1978; Wilcox and Webster, 1980). In the task, a client is engaged in a conversation that is usually 60 minutes in length. During the course of the conversation a clinician pretends to misunderstand the client by asking questions (e.g., "What?"; "What did you say?"; or "Humm?"). The aphasic client's response to these queries is analyzed in order to assess repair strategies. Newhoff and coworkers examined changes clients' made in their original messages following the query. They viewed these changes as repair strategies and classified the repairs in accordance with the following parameters:

1. Complete or partial repetitions of the original message.
2. Linguistic repairs including semantic, syntactic, or phonological changes that occurred without making a significant change in the original meaning.
3. Significant changes in the original meaning that were accomplished through the addition or deletion of information.

The task used by Newhoff and coworkers unquestionably evaluates an aspect of behavior central to aphasic communicative effectiveness, namely, the ability to clarify or repair a misunderstood message. Aphasic clients often are misunderstood, and it is important to evaluate their strategies for dealing with such situations. In their analyses of repair strategies, Newhoff and coworkers primarily focused on verbal behavior. We would additionally recommend that analyses of nonverbal behavior be conducted. Many times an aphasic client can make a nonverbal repair that is more successful than one that is verbal. Additionally, in the clinical application of this task, we would recommend that clinicians avoid using only "What?" or "What did you say?" as the queries. It has been found that these particular queries are most likely to result in a repetition of the original message (Wilcox and Webster, 1980). For this reason, sole use of these queries is likely to yield results not actually representative of the diversity of a client's repair strategies. Examples of other query types include (a) an interrogative repetition of the patient's communicative attempt (e.g., "The paper?"), (b) a puzzled facial expression, and (c) production of a statement requesting more information (e.g., "I don't understand. Can you let me know more?").

We would suggest that in many cases, one may not need to *pretend* to misunderstand an aphasic client. Patients frequently experience communicative breakdowns, and we would recommend that clinicians avoid intentionally exposing their patients to such additional frustration. However, we also recognize that as clinicians become familiar with a client, they may be likely to comprehend messages that would not be comprehended by an unfamiliar listener. When this seems to be the case, a structured task such as the one described is a useful way to evaluate a client's repair strategies.

Role-Playing

Some clinicians have attempted to assess aphasic persons' general communicative effectiveness by engaging them in role-playing activities (e.g., Holland, 1980; Ulatowska, Macaluso-Haynes, and Mendel-Richardson, 1976; Davis and Wilcox, 1981). Typically, in role-playing tasks a common activity is selected (e.g., getting a prescription refilled) and a client is asked to behave and communicate as if the activity were actually occurring. Holland (1980) used role-playing tasks in one portion of the CADL and evaluated clients' communicative behavior by scoring communicative attempts as "correct," "adequate," or "wrong."

Ulatowska and coworkers (1976) conducted role-playing assessments in their clients' homes. They prepared scripts and prompts and asked the asphasic clients to role-play such activities as ordering a meal from a restaurant and paying the bill and depositing checks at a bank. They evaluated communicative effectiveness by noting modalities that were used for communication as well as delays that accompanied communicative efforts.

Davis and Wilcox (1981) described role-playing techniques that could be performed in a clinical setting. They used role-playing assessments primarily as a probe to determine aspects of treatment progress. In their discussion of role-playing batteries, they stressed the importance of selecting activities that included those a patient might actually need to perform (e.g., obtaining assistance from someone). They recommended that the actual activities should include those capable of eliciting communicative strategies applicable to a variety of situations (e.g., requesting information, giving instructions, requesting clarification). Davis and Wilcox constructed a set of situations that included props and a script of prompts to be produced by a clinician. A patient's communicative success was scored in relation to the number of prompts that had to be provided by a clinician prior to message communication. For example, a situation requiring no prompts from a clinician would be regarded as more successful than one that required three prompts from a clinician.

Role-playing techniques can be a useful way of gleaning information as to how an aphasic person may function in situations that cannot be directly observed in a clinical setting. However, some degree of caution should be exerted in generalizing the results to a client's natural communicative abilities. Role-playing tasks are somewhat abstract and may tap abilities more cognitive than communicative in nature, particularly for patients who have global aphasia (Gurland and coworkers, 1982). Furthermore, our experience with role-playing activities has indicated that sometimes it is very difficult for an aphasic person to understand the actual task. We think this may be due to the rather abstract nature of some role-playing activities. Hence, role-playing activities may not be appropriate for more severely impaired aphasic individuals. Finally, role-playing activities, like structured tasks, are rarely suitable as a starting point for pragmatic assessments. A role-playing task is most appropriate to use either as a means of assessing use of strategies that have been identified from other assessments or observations or as a treatment probe to assess aspects of generalization of treatment targets.

Questionnaires

Some use has been made of questionnaires in order to obtain information about an aphasic person's communicative abilities. Ulatowska and coworkers (1976) and Ulatowska, Haynes, Hildebrand, and Richardson (1977) presented questionnaires to aphasic patients, their employers, their family members, and their close friends. Their questionnaire items focused on such areas as (a) speech habits of an aphasic client (e.g., "Does he or she initiate conversation or only respond to others?"), (b) an aphasic person's personal communicative needs (e.g., "Do you handle your own money, write checks, or balance your checkbook?"), and (c) evaluation of an aphasic client's communicative abilities in his or her employment setting (e.g., "How well does he or she give instructions and make explanations to other employees or customers?").

Although questionnaires will not elicit complete information, they are capable of assisting a clinician in gathering general data that may prove useful for determining interests, typical communicative contexts, pre-aphasic speech habits, and potentially desirable and undesirable communicative strategies. Therefore, questionnaires, like structured tasks and role-playing activities, are not appropriate as a single assessment. However, we would recommend that questionnaires be employed in the initial assessment process, because they will provide general information concerning a patient's communicative needs. This informaton will be particularly useful in determining contextual variables that may need to be manipulated in the more complete assessments. For example, if an aphasic client does not handle his or her own money or does not work, there will be no initial need to assess communicative performance in these areas. This is not to say that such areas may not be a latter assessment and treatment focus. Obviously, as recovery progresses, a goal of many treatment programs is to have a person begin resuming his or her pre-aphasic responsibilities.

Natural Observations

Unquestionably, the best way to learn about aphasic clients' everyday communicative abilities is to observe them as they go about their daily routines. Holland (1982) has described a system for observing aphasic persons in their natural environments. The observational categories she used for field visits are as follows:

1.   Verbal Output
     a. Form—verbal lubricant, social conventions, asks questions, makes requests, answers questions and requests, volunteers information
     b. Style—agrees, disagrees, teases, uses humor, sarcasm, or metaphor
     c. Conversational dominance—interrupts or changes topics
     d. Correctional strategies—corrects, clarifies, requests
     e. Metalinguistics—comments on own speaking, responds to phonemic cues
2.   Nonverbal Output—spatial indicators, gestures to maintain conversation, humor, and affective states
3.   Read/Write/Math—responds to written material, writing, responds to numbers
4.   Other—talks on phone, talks to pets, talks to self, responds to household sounds, sings, speaks in a foreign language

Although Holland (1980) had previously reported that 60 minute observations constitute a representative sample, in this field technique observations were conducted for a period of two hours. An observer simply "followed a patient around" and tallied occurrences of the behavior of interest in terms of success or failure. Successes and failures were defined as follows: "Any observed response that communicated the aphasic patient's message was considered to be successful, regardless of the means used to convey it. Conversely, any response that did not succeed in communicating the aphasic person's message, regardless of the means used, was considered a failure" (p. 50).

Natural observations, like conversational samples or formal tests, constitute an excellent pragmatic assessment. Of all pragmatic procedures, natural observations yield the most representative information and, as such, are probably the most useful for planning and conducting treatment. In a field observation a clinician has the unique opportunity to determine a patient's important contextual parameters, their overall communicativeness, and particular communicative strategies that are successful as well as unsuccessful. This information can then be used to determine treatment content in the form of communicative strategies to establish, to enhance, and to de-emphasize.

RECOMMENDATIONS FOR PRAGMATIC ASSESSMENT

Thus far, we have considered issues concerning appropriate content as well as a variety of procedures that may be used for pragmatic assessments. We have emphasized the dual face of pragmatic assessments, that is, a focus upon the identification of pragmatic strengths and limitations and a focus upon determining a patient's overall communicative effectiveness. Not all pragmatic assessment approaches are appropriate for all types and levels of aphasia, nor can all be viewed as feasible, given the varying work settings and time limitations of clinical aphasiologists. Within the limitations of patient and clinical characteristics, it is important to select an assessment approach that will yield representative information concerning an aphasic person's communicative strategies. We generally can say that the selection and administration of assessments is governed by three variables. These include (a) the capacity of a given instrument for identifying an aphasic person's natural communicative strategies, (b) the severity of aphasic impairment, and (c) the work setting and time constraints of the clinical aphasiologist.

Identifying Communicative Strategies

Some pragmatic techniques will yield an overall index of communicative functioning (e.g., CADL; FCP; Prutting and Kirchner Pragmatic Checklist, 1983) whereas other techniques will give more specific information concerning communicative strategies (e.g., turn-taking, repair strategies, contingent queries). As we have previously mentioned, both approaches may be important for the treatment process. It is important to gain an overall understanding of an aphasic client's communicative abilities. It is equally important to identify the various strategies he or she may be using as a means of compensating for the aphasic impairment. Some strategies may be helpful for the communication process whereas others may inhibit or hinder communication. Knowledge of the particular strategies an aphasic person has developed is important for purposes of treatment planning and implementation.

Several of the techniques discussed in the previous section of this chapter are suitable for purposes of identifying an aphasic person's communicative strategies. In general, regardless of the analysis system to be used, we believe an assessment should begin with the aphasiologist obtaining some sort of conversational sample. Types of conversational samples as well as methods of obtaining them were discussed earlier in this chapter. We recommend that the clinician obtain a spontaneous conversational sample. We recognize that in some cases a newly aphasic client may be reluctant to initiate spontaneous communicative interactions, and a clinical aphasiologist may have to rely on elicitation procedures in order to obtain an adequate sample. We also recommend that several different samples on subsequent days and in different contexts be obtained. In many cases, contextual conditions will have a significant effect on communicative behavior. Thus repeated measures are necessary in order to ensure a degree of representativeness of an assessment. Finally, if possible, a sample should be videotaped. In this way it can be reviewed several times, and many nonverbal strategies can be easily identified. If videotaping is not possible, then the clinician can employ an audiotape and supplement his or her observations by using a tally sheet in which behavior is categorized (e.g., pantomime, gesticulations) and frequency of occurrence is noted.

After samples have been obtained, we recommend analyzing them to obtain a record of successful versus unsuccessful communicative attempts (e.g., Holland, 1982). This record may be an index of behaviors associated with successful and unsuccessful communicative attempts. To accomplish this indexing, an aphasiologist may choose to rely on systems developed by other clinicians (e.g., Holland, 1982; Prutting and Kirchner, 1983; the guidelines presented in Tables 3-1 and 3-2), or he or she may prefer to review the sample and create new categories. The end result of this indexing should be a comprehensive list of an aphasic person's communicative strategies in a variety of contexts. It is highly probable that the success of a strategy will vary as a function of such factors as the communicative participants, the purpose of the communicative interaction, and the setting of the interaction. Further, it is likely that some strategies will be identified that are successful across contexts. Not only does such information serve as important baseline data but it also proves invaluable for treatment planning, an issue which is considered in more detail in Chapters 4 and 5.

Severity of Aphasic Impairment

The severity of aphasic impairment may influence the particular assessment techniques and goals. Both of the formal tests discussed in the previous section as well as the more globally oriented indices of communicative behavior (e.g., Gurland et al., 1982; Houghton et al., 1982; Prutting and Kirchner, 1983) are appropriate for most levels of aphasic impairment. However, special considerations may be necessary when dealing with severely and mildly involved clients.

Although we generally have concluded that most aphasic clients have relatively intact pragmatic abilities, clients with severe global aphasia may represent a group with which the clinical aphasiologist might expect numerous pragmatic as well as symbolic deficits. Such expectations should be reflected in the choice of assessment procedures. With these types of clients it may be important initially to obtain an index of appropriate versus inappropriate pragmatic behaviors. The pragmatic checklist developed by Prutting and Kirchner (1983) should serve this purpose well. The CCEI (Houghton et al., 1982) may also be useful for globally impaired patients, because it evaluates such parameters as responses to speech and gross environmental sounds. In general, assessment approaches with severely impaired patients should include those that evaluate nonverbal aspects of pragmatic behavior (e.g., expression of affect, use of facial expressions, turn-taking ability). That is not to say that one should avoid evaluation of linguistic strategies. This sort of evaluation can certainly be attempted. Bond, Ulatowska, Macaluso-Haynes, and May (1983) reported that, when attempts were made to elicit narrative discourse from severely involved patients, they retained the intent tell a story but could not produce the discourse elements. Because many globally impaired patients are largely nonverbal, a linguistically oriented assessment focus may not yield a great deal of information and, in some cases, could hinder identification of effective communicative strategies.

Aphasic clients demonstrating mild impairment also require specialized assessment procedures. In many cases repeated samples with varying contexts are necessary in order to obtain an accurate picture of communicative functioning. Such persons may function very well in most contextual conditions and demonstrate problems in only a few selected conditions. It is the responsibility of the clinical aphasiologist to identify such conditions in the client's environment in order to effectively plan treatment. Sometimes mildly impaired persons may function acceptably in terms of conveying their messages, but they may be dissatisfied with their performance in situations calling for complex communicative skills or more abstract communicative skills such as metaphor or humor. In these cases some of the more sophisticated analysis techniques may be appropriate (e.g., discourse cohesion abilities, comprehension and expression of humor, comprehension and expression of subtle speaker meaning). For techniques to accomplish such analyses, structured tasks may frequently be appropriate.

Work Settings and Time Constraints

The work settings and time constraints of a clinical aphasiologist are important considerations in the selection of a pragmatic assessment procedure. Such limitations are frequently overlooked by persons advocating management procedures for handicapped individuals. However, we do believe this to be an important consideration. Fortunately, with the variety of assessment approaches available, we believe that adequate representative assessments can be obtained under a variety of working conditions.

Generally, aphasic clients are seen in an acute care facility, a rehabilitation center, or in their homes or nursing homes. For clients seen in an acute care facility, it is practical to conduct primarily general assessments geared toward identifying general level of aphasic impairment. Such initial information then proves useful for the aphasiologist who is responsible for long-term communicative rehabilitation.

For clients who are seen on a continuing basis, more detailed assessments are appropriate. Probably the most ideal setting for obtaining a representative communicative assessment is available to those clinicians involved in home or nursing home care. These settings are ideal, because the client can be observed in his or her natural environment. For these cases, Holland's (1982) field observation system should be quite useful. The procedure requires no specialized equipment (e.g., video or audio recording). Rather, it simply requires tallies of a given client's successful versus unsuccessful communicative behavior in accordance with verbal and nonverbal categories. Further, since these observations are made while the aphasic person is engaging in his or her daily activities, representativeness is almost certain.

Aphasiologists who are not able to observe their clients in their natural environments need to rely on procedures other than field observations. Initially, in order to obtain a picture of communicative functioning outside of the clinical setting, questionnaires may be appropriate. In addition to these, spontaneous (if possible) conversational samples should be obtained with the clinician as well as other persons. Other potential communicative participants include a family member, another clinician, and other aphasic clients. Finally, structured tasks or role-playing activities can be used to assess general effectiveness of communicative strategies or use of a particular communicative strategy.

Many of the assessment techniques we have described take time. When time spent in such assessments is added to other standardized measures, it initially may appear excessive, and in fact, we would caution aphasiologists against "overassessment." Typically, one global measure, accompanied by an analysis of "suspect" features should suffice. Although we have discussed aspects of pragmatic assessment in terms of initial evaluations, many evaluation techniques can and should be accomplished as a part of the treatment process (e.g., structured tasks, role-playing) in which the focus is upon remediation as well as evaluation. In the next chapter we shall discuss one way of using a technique for eliciting conversation (e.g., picture description when a picture is hidden from view of a listener) in order to construct a treatment program. Finally, in many treatment programs, assessment is an ongoing process and many of the techniques we have described can be used as probes to assess treatment progress.

Chapter 4

Incorporating Conversation Structure in Treatment: PACE

The technique called Promoting Aphasics' Communicative Effectiveness (PACE) was introduced in 1978 by Wilcox and Davis in a miniseminar at the annual convention of the American Speech-Language-Hearing Association. It was intended to reshape structured interaction between clinicians and aphasic clients into a form resembling face-to-face conversation. After successfully implementing this new procedure with a variety of aphasic individuals, an instructional videotape was produced (Wilcox and Davis, 1979) and a description of the procedure was published (Davis and Wilcox, 1981). PACE allows for several pragmatic components of communication to occur repeatedly in a standard clinical environment. These components include an expression of a wide range of speech acts, turn-taking between participants, hint-and-guess sequences when communication breakdown occurs, opportunities to make use of variables governing expression and comprehension of given and new information, and opportunities to make use of linguistic, paralinguistic, and extralinguistic contexts. We approach our discussion of PACE initially by describing the overall treatment interaction. Following this, we consider each of the treatment principles and their rationales in some detail. We conclude by considering issues relative to the implementation and measurement of PACE and PACE-related activities as a function of the varying types and levels of aphasic impairment.

Procedures in PACE are based upon four principles, each of which are characteristic of processes occurring in natural communicative settings. The specific principles are as follows:

1. The clinician and client participate equally as sender and receiver of messages.

2. The treatment interaction consists of an exchange of new information between clinician and client.
3. The client is allowed free choice with respect to selection of communicative channels with which to convey messages.
4. Feedback from the clinician is based on the client's success in communicating a message and is characteristic of receiver feedback occurring in natural settings.

The PACE procedure employs a structured core activity on which many variations are possible. In this core activity the clinician and client(s) are seated at a table, and a stack of stimulus items is placed face down in the middle of the table and within easy reach of all participants. These stimulus items, which can be pictured or written, serve as topics for a series of brief conversations that take place in the interaction. The basic task is for each participant (clinician and client) to take turns selecting a stimulus topic, keeping it hidden from view of the other participant, and communicating information about the topic such that the participant can guess what is represented on the stimulus card.

In the PACE activity the principal objective of the participants is to communicate a particular message. The clinical objective is to improve clients' symbolic abilities that are utilized to convey the messages. Thus, the primary focus of the treatment is on a given client's communicative, as opposed to symbolic, adequacy. In meeting the PACE objectives each participant assumes basic roles of sender and receiver. The aphasic person is assumed to be able to utilize certain components, such as his or her pragmatic knowledge concerning conversational functioning, and is also expected to draw on a variety of channels to communicate a particular message.

We believe that the PACE approach is appropriate as a treatment task for all types and levels of aphasia. Our basic assumption is that any aphasic individual can communicate in some way. In meeting the requirement of appropriateness many variations can be applied to the core activity in order to ensure its suitability for each aphasic person. The variations may be in the form of stimulus changes, although adjustments can also be made with respect to response expectations. These issues are considered more specifically in later sections of this chapter. At this time we want to focus upon presenting a step-by-step implementation of the PACE principles. Although we shall discuss these principles separately, we want to remind our readers that in reality the principles are interdependent. Hence, we believe that the most effective treatment interaction results from the combinatory effects of the principles.

EQUAL PARTICIPATION

The first principle of PACE concerns the level of participation by the clinician and client. The clinician and aphasic person participate equally as senders and receivers of messages by taking turns or alternating in communicating messages about the stimulus items to each other. This principle sets the overall tone for the PACE interaction and, in doing such, allows the clinician and client the opportunity to engage in a communicative interaction in accordance with turn-taking conventions as described in Chapter 1.

The turn-taking occurring in PACE can be described at two levels. The first pertains to topic initiation and response sequences. When the clinician selects the stimulus item, he or she can be viewed as the topic initiator while the client can be regarded as the topic responder. Conversely, when the client selects a stimulus item, he or she becomes the topic initiator while the clinician serves as respondent. Thus, at one level we can say that the clinician and aphasic client take turns serving as initiators and responders of topics. However, turn-taking also occurs within each initiation and response sequence with the possibility of several turns being exchanged over the same topic as in the following example:

> Client: (picks up card, stands up and gestures with both hands making a motion resembling digging)
> Clinician: Shoveling?
> Client: No.
> Clinician: Sweeping?
> Client: Yes.
> Clinician: (to confirm) Sweeping?
> Client: Yes, there it is (shows card).
> Clinician: She's sweeping the kitchen floor. Right?
> Client: That's right.

In the preceding example, we would describe the client as the topic initiator. However, in the process of communicating the message he served as a sender as well as receiver. Thus, in PACE, turn-taking can be conceptualized at two levels. The first is more global and pertains to topic initiation versus responding to a topic initiated by the participant. The second level concerns the exchange of turns while communicating about a specific topic. Overall we can say that the equal participation principle accomplishes three important goals: (a) It allows the aphasic client experience with topic or turn initiation or sending as well as topic or turn responses; (b) it allows the clinician to serve as a model for initiation and sending as well as responding and thereby provides opportunities for the clinician to emphasize or de-emphasize communicative channels; and (c) it allows the aphasic client to gain experience sustaining a communicative interaction for several turns over the same topic.

The Aphasic Client: Initiator and Respondent

Within each of these roles aphasic persons have the opportunity to develop and use several important communicative strategies. As an *initiator*, several types of pragmatic behavior are required. First, the context (linguistic, paralinguistic, and extralinguistic) must be considered so that an appropriate and relevant message is formulated. In considering contexts clients rely on their knowledge of prior as well as current contextual information, such as conceptual knowledge they may share with their clinicians about a certain topic as well as environmental contextual cues that may influence message transmission comprehension. Thus, as topic initiators clients will need to discern what need not be restated, because it is already known, as well as what needs to be stated in order for the message to be comprehensible.

Following these initial contextual considerations a client may need to obtain a clinician's attention through appropriate verbal (e.g., saying his or her name) or nonverbal (e.g., eye contact) conventions. Additional communicative strategies required of the client pertain to symbol selection. Specifically, the symbolic means used to produce a message must be in accordance with rules concerning given and new distinctions, and the message must also be constructed such that it is in accordance with the intended intent (e.g., request, statement, question).

The final communicative strategy required of the aphasic person, when serving as initiator, relates to ambiguous messages. If the respondent (clinician) indicates a lack of understanding, the original initiator (aphasic client) should be able to repair the turn. In an attempt to repair a turn, the aphasic person will need to apply the clinician feedback to his or her original message and provide a reformulated message. Thus an aphasic person is required to engage in a self-monitoring process through this form of message comparison and evaluation.

When an aphasic client is serving as *respondent*, a different set of communicative behaviors is required. Generally these are based upon receptive processes, but certain expressive behavior may also be necessary. Receptively, a client is required to decode the relevant contextual information and also apply given and new conventions to the message that is received. Once the initiator has completed transmission of the message, an aphasic client should then provide feedback. The feedback may be in the form of a response indicating what message was received (e.g., "I understand, you're talking about a horse," or "Are you describing a horse?"), or it may be a contingent query or clarification request (e.g., "I'm not sure, something about a horse?"). Thus the aphasic person is also required to engage in self-monitoring of receptive processes by evaluating his or her message comprehension and providing the appropriate form of feedback.

The Clinician: A Model for Initiating/Sending and Receiving

A clinician, when serving in each of these roles, is also serving as a communicative model. Through appropriate use of modeling a clinician may modify an aphasic client's communicative behavior. Desirable communicative behavior can be strengthened or established while undesirable behavior can be minimized or eliminated. The theoretical basis for modeling is drawn from social learning theory (Bandura and Harris, 1966) and has been widely applied in the area of child language development and disorders (Orazi and Wilcox, 1982; Wilcox, 1984; Wilcox and Leonard, 1978). Thus the effectiveness of modeling as a clinical procedure has a sound theoretical as well as research base.

Overall, a clinician uses his or her modeling role as an opportunity to reinforce a client's communicative capabilities as well as to demonstrate use of particular communicative strategies. The types of behavior being modeled by a clinician then influence a client's communicative behavior. It is important to note that a clinician influences, not directs, a client's communicative behavior. In PACE, and in the application of the equal participation principle in particular, an aphasic person is never directly instructed by a clinician to use a particular communicative channel. A patient always has free choice with respect to selection of communicative channels. Change is established in a patient's use of particular communicative strategies as a function of the influences associated with clinician modeling.

Basically, when a clinician is serving as topic initiator or sender, he or she should employ communicative strategies that are desirable for the aphasic patient to use when it is his or her turn to serve as topic initiator or sender. When a clinician is serving as respondent (i.e., a client is the topic initiator or sender), he or she would respond with communicative strategies that are desirable for the aphasic client to use in the respondent role. Our clinical observation has been that clinicians' initiating or sending behavior influences that same behavior in clients, while clinicians' respondent behavior influences responding behavior in clients. Although additional research is required to substantiate the notion, this means that a clinician's initiation or sending behavior may have minimal effect on a client's communicative strategies used to respond to messages. In the same way a clinician's response to a client's message may have minimal impact on communicative strategies used by a client to send messages.

In order to illustrate this relationship of clinician behavior to client behavior, we shall describe an exemplary treatment session with an aphasic client who demonstrated limited verbal skills and relatively poor auditory comprehension. The goals were to increase the client's verbal functioning with respect to sending messages and to improve her verbal comprehension when receiving messages. The clinician sent primarily verbal messages as an attempt to model the target sending behavior. A nonverbal response was required when the client was serving as receiver (e.g., pointing to a picture that corresponded to the clinician's message) because her relatively poor auditory comprehension created uncertainty as to whether she actually comprehended the clinician's verbal messages. Thus the clinician functioned as a verbal sender and a nonverbal receiver. Analysis of a series of treatment sessions revealed that the majority of the time (approximately 89 per cent) the client sent messages in the verbal channel and received messages by pointing to a picture.

As an additional example, let us consider clinician modeling in a client who feels the need to constantly verbalize, particularly as a respondent, thereby experiencing difficulty comprehending conversational interactions. This would resemble the sort of client described in the literature as demonstrating "press for speech," a phenomenon creating particular difficulty with comprehension. A goal with such a client might be to decrease use of verbal behavior when receiving messages in order to create a situation more conducive to comprehension. Because it is likely that a clinician's receiving behavior (versus sending behavior) will have the most impact on a client's receiving behavior, a clinician might choose to be a nonverbal respondent by pointing to a picture as a means of confirming understanding of a message. The aphasic client then has the opportunity to observe the clinician receiving messages without verbalizing and, as was discussed in a previous example, may also begin receiving messages nonverbally.

As a further example, let us consider a client who has an extremely poor prognosis for verbal recovery yet still insists on primary use of the verbal modality for sending messages. A goal with such a client would probably be to increase use of more effective communicative modalities. An initial step in accomplishing this goal focuses upon clinician behavior when serving as a sender of messages. It would be important for a clinician to begin modeling such things as use of extralinguistic (e.g., gestures, writing, facial expressions) and paralinguistic cues to supplement verbal information.

As a final example, we shall consider clients who may pretend to comprehend a message when they are serving as a receiver. Clinical experience has indicated that such clients are identifiable from situations resembling the following:

> The clinician has just sent a message, the client may respond with "Oh yes, right," and the clinician may interpret this as accurate comprehension and show the client his or her card. Upon seeing the card the client might say something like "Oh, that one." Or perhaps the client points to a picture to indicate message reception and points to a picture that does not correspond to the clinician's message. Although in the second instance the clinician can readily identify miscomprehension, the common factor in both examples is lack of client comprehension.

One desirable communicative strategy for such clients might be to increase their use of contingent queries when they are serving as receivers of messages. To accomplish this, the clinician, when serving as a receiver, may wish to make a special point of producing contingent queries. It is likely with many aphasic persons that the clinician will be modeling such behavior anyway. That is, when providing feedback, the clinician will certainly experience many instances in which he or she will not fully comprehend a client's message. What we are suggesting is that if a clinician is working with a client who makes little use of contingent queries, then their appropriate use should be emphasized in the PACE interaction.

The Aphasic Client: Sustaining a Topic

We have previously described the two levels of turn-taking inherent in the equal participation principle. Thus far we have focused only on the more global turn level. We shall now turn our attention to the exchange of turns with a given stimulus or topic item. Within the framework of trying to convey a particular message, the clinician and client, regardless of who served as the original initiator or sender, may take several mini-turns as sender and receiver of messages about the same topic. This mini-turn sequence allows the client to coordinate his or her symbolic functioning (both receptively and expressively) with several pragmatic behaviors. First, the symbolic devices important for the distinction of given versus new information may be employed. These include ellipses, use of definite and indefinite articles, initialization, pronominalization, and stress manipulation. Second, the client has the opportunity to make use of turn-taking conventions that are important for sustaining an interaction on a particular topic. These conventions include relatedness of turns, confirmation of received communications, production of contingent queries, repair of turns, and minimal overlap of turns.

As with the global turn sequence (i.e., alternating selection of stimulus cards) the clinician has the opportunity to serve as a model for all of these communicative behaviors involved in sustaining an interaction around a given topic. In order to illustrate clinician modeling as well as client opportunities to use various pragmatic strategies, the reader is referred to a scripted segment of a PACE interaction (Table 4-1).

In this sample script, which represents a mini-turn sequence, the pragmatic behavior demonstrated by each person is in brackets. Initially the client specified the topic. The clinician then produced a contingent query and also used the definite article to signal given information. The client then attempted to repair the turn and employed pronominalization, another device used to indicate given information. The clinician produced a second contingent query and also used pronominalization. The client then confirmed this message, and the clinician followed this with an additional confirmation.

In this example the client used pragmatically appropriate strategies. The clinician can be viewed as modeling use of contingent queries as well as ellipsis. If the client had not used various strategies, then the clinician would have wanted to model desirable options. For example, let's say the client's response to the clinician's contingent query was "A woman," plus the writing gesture. The clinician's same response ("Oh, she's writing") would have served as a model for the use of pronominalization.

We would like to mention that failure to comply with certain pragmatic strategies involving symbols does not generally result in inadequate messages. For example, a failure by a client to use pronominalization does not significantly affect message comprehension by a receiver. Although the primary goal of PACE is to give a client experience with communicating adequate messages, a secondary focus is placed upon improving the use of symbols to do such. Thus, a clinician's modeling of particular symbolic devices within a turn sequence can be viewed in a dual manner. First, it is a response to the communicative adequacy of a message and, second, it provides a normal model of symbol use.

EXCHANGE OF NEW INFORMATION

As discussed in Chapter 1, communication generally occurs between persons as a means of exchanging new information. Such information can

Table 4-1.   Example of a Mini-Turn Sequence in a PACE Interaction

Client: (picks up a card) "A woman. . . paper."
Clinician: "A woman with the paper?" [contingent query, use of definite article to signal
    given information]
Client: "No, she's. . ." (makes writing gesture). [pronominalization, repair]
Clinician: "Oh, she's writing?" [pronominalization, contingent query]
Client: "Yes." (shows card) [confirmation]
Clinician: "She's writing." [confirmation]

Brackets indicate the pragmatic behavior of each participant.

be in the form of ideas or beliefs that are an expansion of shared information, or it may be an introduction of entirely new ideas. In a sense, communicative interactions can be conceptualized as a pyramid, the base of which is regarded as shared knowledge. Unless there is a need for re-emphasis or review, communicators do not need to reiterate the base information. Rather, they provide additional information that either relates to or enhances the base knowledge.

There are a number of conversational conventions to follow with respect to the expression of given versus new information (e.g., ellipsis, pronominalization). These conventions serve as assumptions, or shared knowledge, for all communicators as they are engaging in conversations. Thus, let's consider an example where two people are looking at a picture of a hippopotamus. In this case there is no need for one person to say "That's a hippo," since that is information readily available to both people. Appropriate comments in this particular context would be such things as opinions ("That's a large hippo"), feelings ("I really like hippos"), or informative statements ("I have six hippos at home").

Many treatment protocols for aphasic individuals are structured such that the communicative participants are not making use of conversational rules governing given versus new information. For example, in many procedures a clinician might show a client a picture and ask him or her to either name or describe the picture. The crucial feature here is that the picture is in view of both the clinician and client. Therefore, the verbalization represents information already shared by both participants. In the PACE procedure we are interested in avoiding a redundant situation such as this. Thus we attempt to create a context that is conducive to reliance on rules governing conveyance of new and given information.

An attempt is made to create the "new information" principle in PACE by having the initiator or sender keep his or her message stimulus hidden from view of the receiver. As explained in the overview, this is accomplished by having a single stack of stimuli that are placed face down on a table. Thus, the perceived goal of each participant, when serving as topic initiator or sender, is to transmit a message that is not known to the receiver.

Because a clinician selects the conversational stimuli before a treatment session, he or she may be able to anticipate the nature of a message to be conveyed before the client has in fact sent sufficient information. This may be particularly true if the same stimuli are used repeatedly. This factor reduces the extent to which the new information principle can be applied in reality. This concern was addressed by Davis (1980) as a problem area with the PACE procedure. We believe that this difficulty can be minimized if a large number of stimuli are used and the stimuli are changed frequently. Stimuli may be chosen by a third party, such as another clinician, a secretary, or a spouse. Finally, if no other avenues are available, a clinician may need to do some "pretending" about his or her awareness of the nature of stimuli. However, this sort of pretending can be very unnatural for a clinician as well as a patient and should be avoided whenever possible.

FREE CHOICE OF COMMUNICATIVE CHANNELS

This principle pertains primarily to an aphasic person's sending behavior. In natural face-to-face interactions, senders have a variety of means that can be utilized in order to convey messages (Harrison, 1974). Such channels can include the use of verbal, graphic, or gestural behaviors (see Chapter 3). In order to incorporate this aspect of natural conversation into the PACE interaction, aphasic clients are allowed to select the communicative channel(s) with which to convey their messages.

By including the element of free choice in PACE, we are essentially following the recommendations of Holland (1977), in which she suggested that aphasic clients be allowed to use any available means for purposes of message transmission. Her recommendations came in part from the observation that frequently in aphasia treatment there is more focus on symbolic perfection than communicative adequacy. This concern was also addressed by Wilcox and Davis (1977), who suggested that in many cases aphasic persons are focused on linguistic perfection to the extent that they may inadvertently limit their communicative effectiveness. Thus, the free choice option in PACE is intended to provide clients with the opportunity to exercise effective communicative strategies that need not always be verbal in nature. Essentially clients discover that existing abilities do indeed convey new information and that new abilities may also arise within the interaction.

The inclusion of such an option is not intended to minimize the importance of focusing treatment upon the development of effective linguistic expression. Indeed, in many cases it will be desirable to focus upon linguistic expression during treatment. Furthermore, the principle of free choice extends to *choice of linguistic surface structure* to convey an idea. For example, time may be expressed with an adverb (e.g., "I go Wednesday again"), and a question may be expressed with syntax (e.g., "Is she done?") or intonation (e.g., "She done?"). By allowing the clients free choice in PACE, the treatment focus is placed upon communicative adequacy and upon symbolic choice in achieving communicative adequacy.

In implementing the free choice principle, a clinician should remember that an aphasic client is not directly instructed to use a particular channel. Rather, the clinician influences channel usage by modeling desirable channels when he or she is serving as sender. Also, a client may happen upon or self-generate a strategy that works for communication. The client thereby engages in a self-discovery process as to effective communicative options or channels. This discovery process is facilitated by the feedback principle that is discussed in the next section of this chapter. What is important for the moment is that many patients may be more likely to continue using strategies of their own choosing rather than strategies that a clinician tells them to use.

As a clinician is structuring the PACE interaction it is important that he or she create an atmosphere in which the client understands that conveying his or her message, even though there may be symbolic imperfections, is the primary goal of treatment. Further, the clinician should make sure that the client realizes that there is a choice as to how the message can be transmitted. The aphasic person's awareness of these two factors can be facilitated by using instructions something like the following in the initiation of a PACE activity:

> We are going to take turns letting each other know what is on these cards. Our goal is going to be for each of us to guess what is on each other's card. I would like for you to start by picking a card and not letting me see it. Then, let me know what is on the card in any way you can without actually showing it to me.

Although the preceding instructions will serve as a starting point, many clients may initially attempt to verbalize. It is therefore up to the clinician to immediately model the goal of communicating messages in any possible manner. Furthermore, it is up to the clinician to demonstrate that the *primary* focus is upon effective communication, not the means by which such effectiveness is achieved. Additionally, with some clients (e.g., those with significant auditory comprehension deficits) it may be best for the clinician to begin the interaction by taking two or three turns and then indicating that it is the client's turn.

It is important for clinicians to realize, and clients to learn, that messages can be transmitted effectively with a variety of channels. A clinician needs to make sure that opportunities are provided to use various channels by making appropriate materials available (e.g., paper, pencil, pictures, alphabet cards, word lists). The type, level, and number of channels to be made available will vary as a function of a particular client's unique abilities and needs and should include those that a client will be likely to use outside the clinical setting. Potential channels might include speaking, writing, gestures, pointing to printed words, drawing a picture, or pointing to related pictures. Frequently messages may be expressed via notebooks that aphasic clients can carry with them for facilitation of message transmission. If such notebooks are already being used by a client, they should be incorporated into a PACE activity. If such materials are introduced in PACE, they initially may not be as convenient or portable as desirable. Thus an eventual goal for some clients might be the creation and use of notebook materials that are convenient and practical for real life.

Many communicative channels can function effectively in combinations, and sometimes the most effective message transmission may be such channel combinations. Frequently, a verbalization or a gesture in isolation may not get a message across, but a combination of the two accomplishes that end. Davis and Wilcox (1981) reported an example of such combinatory behavior with a client demonstrating Wernicke's aphasia: he conveyed the message *tree* by pointing to a potted plant and saying "almost." Thus, a clinician should remember the communicative potential of combinations and be sure to model potentially effective channel combinations when serving as sender.

FEEDBACK BASED ON COMMUNICATIVE ADEQUACY

PACE has thus far been described as a procedure in which (a) the clinician and aphasic client alternate as message senders, (b) the sender uses any channel that maximizes success in communicating a message, and (c) the message to be communicated is known only to the sender. The fourth principle concerns a clinician's role as receiver when an aphasic client is serving as sender. When a clinician is serving as receiver, he or she provides feedback that is based upon a client's success in communicating a message. Irrespective of the communicative channel utilized, a client is considered to have communicated successfully if the clinician comprehends the message.

The form of clinician feedback provided in PACE differs from feedback that is commonly provided in aphasia treatment. That is, in many other forms of treatment interaction, clinician feedback involves immediate positive reinforcement and the encouragement of linguistically adequate responses. When a response falls short of a defined criterion, a cue is usually provided so as to improve a client's response. Cuing is possible because a clinician knows what a client is supposed to be saying, and often the client is supposed to be saying one particular thing. Cues may consist of an initial sound, a carrier phrase, a printed word, or a spoken model of the word to be repeated by the client. In PACE, this form of clinician feedback is modified so as to focus less on the specific symbolic means used to convey a message and more on comprehension of message content. For the most part, traditional cuing is impossible, since a clinician should not know exactly what a client is trying to convey.

As in most approaches to treatment, feedback in PACE occurs immediately following a client's communication. The specific form of clinician feedback is initially contingent upon the communicative adequacy of an aphasic client's message. That is, a clinician responds to that which he or she has comprehended and, in doing so, provides feedback that resembles reciprocal interactions occurring in *natural conversation.* A clinician's comprehension may be total, partial, or absent. The specific feedback provided by a clinician will relate to (a) the degree of comprehension, which is a function of a client's message adequacy, and (b) a given clinician's receiving style.

For example, let us consider an aphasic client who attempts to convey the concept of reading a newspaper and does such with a precise gesture indicating turning of pages and says "paper." In this case a clinician would probably understand the message and might respond with "I understand, you mean reading a newspaper" or "Oh, do you mean reading a newspaper?" Although both forms of feedback indicate understanding, one is in the form of a statement to be confirmed or disconfirmed, whereas the other is in the form of a hypothesis or question to be confirmed or disconfirmed.

When a clinician/receiver is faced with a more ambiguous message, the feedback may indicate partial understanding or a complete lack of understanding. In many cases the amount of information conveyed via clinician feedback is a combination of the client's message adequacy as well as the clinician's normal receiving style. For example, let us consider the same example of a client who is required to convey the concept of reading a newspaper and does so by moving his or her head from right to left. Some clinicians may have no idea as to the message and respond with "I don't understand, can you let me know more?" Feedback of this sort provides very little information about why the communication was ambiguous; it is simply a statement informing the client that the message was not received. Some clinicians in the same situation may provide more informative feedback, even though they may be equally as puzzled with the initial communication. This more informative feedback may take the form of providing a guess as in "I'm not sure. You're looking at something?" This type of feedback, which is usually in a question (i.e., guess) format, provides a client with more information relative to what he or she may have originally conveyed.

To a certain extent the ability to provide a guess is related to the client's message adequacy, with the assumption being that something informative must be conveyed in order to formulate a guess. However, the degree of information required, in order for clinicians or receivers to make a guess, varies as a function of the individual receiver. Some people may be able to formulate a guess based on little information; while others may require more. It is likely that the ability to guess is related to the listener's attention to the speaker as well as familiarity with an aphasic client or the topic.

One of our recommendations concerning receiver feedback is for clinicians to attempt to provide guesses when they are faced with ambiguous messages. It would appear that a guess, because it does provide more information about a communicative attempt, might facilitate a patient's attempt to make an adequate message repair. At the very least, a guess provides a client with an initial focus for comparison and modification. For example, let us consider the following:

> Client: (selects a card with a picture of a man shaving) Moves her right
> arm up and down approximately 10 inches from her jaw.
> Clinician: "I'm not sure, something about painting?"

In this example the clinician has provided a guess. The client can use this guess by comparing it with her intended message and attempting to make repairs in order to eliminate an interpretation of shaving as painting. On the other hand, if the clinician had provided feedback such as "I don't know," then the client would have had less information to guide her message repair.

Our second recommendation concerning receiving behavior is that whenever possible, a clinician should initially respond with the same channel a client used to send a message. In this way a client has the opportunity to evaluate effectiveness of the channel selected. However, it is also important to remember that the clinician is serving as a model for ideal receiving behavior. In many cases a client's *sending* strategies are not the most desirable *receiving* strategies. Thus, a clinician may also want to provide feedback that models a particular receiving behavior. In such instances it may be that the channels modeled by a clinician serving as receiver were not used by an aphasic person to send a message. Overall, we would recommend accomplishing optimal receiver feedback in the following way: Initially, the clinician should imitate the client's message (either partially or totally), then he or she should provide what is regarded as the ideal receiver feedback.

In order to illustrate the optimal approach to provision of feedback, we shall again consider a patient demonstrating "press for speech" to the extent that it significantly interferes with comprehension. With such a client one may wish to limit use of verbal behavior to sending messages. Therefore a clinician would want to model verbal sending behavior and nonverbal receiving behavior. However, in keeping with our second recommendation concerning feedback, a clinician would also want to provide feedback using channels the patient employed for sending a message. The task becomes one of providing feedback concerning channel effectiveness while also modeling desirable receiving strategies. The following example illustrates one means of accomplishing both of these goals:

> Client: "It's a, yes, one of those things a something a pen."
> Clinician: "Pen." (points to picture of a pen)

In the example the clinician provided feedback in the channel selected by the patient (i.e., verbal), but in keeping with the goal for the patient's receiving behavior, the verbal feedback was abbreviated and a nonverbal response was employed.

As a further example, let us again consider the client who provides a precise gesture indicating page turning and says "paper." Furthermore, let us say that a desirable receiving behavior for that client is use of a notebook. The clinician would initially imitate the client's message by reproducing the gesture and saying "paper?" After this, she or he would model the target receiving behavior by pointing to the word *newspaper* in the client's notebook. In this way a clinician accomplishes the goal of providing same channel feedback and also modeling receiving behavior appropriate for that patient.

The initial provision of imitative feedback is particularly important with ambiguous client messages. With such messages, a clinician initially imitates the ambiguous communication and then, if possible, attempts to formulate a guess, using the channel that would be desirable for the client to use in the receiving role. This can be regarded as the ideal form of feedback for ambiguous communications, because the client has an opportunity to examine his or her actual communicative channel use and then compare that with the guess provided by the clinician.

Another issue affecting clinician receiving behavior concerns those instances in which a client indicates the clinician has comprehended the message when in reality she or he has not. The following sequence would constitute such a situation:

> Client: (selects a picture) "Man. . . yard. . . uh. . . grass, yes, grass"
> Clinician: "A man and grass. Planting? Is he planting grass?"
> Client: "Yes. That's right." (shows picture of a man mowing the lawn)

In this example the client conveyed only partial information but informed the clinician that she had comprehended the entire message. When such instances occur, it is critical for the clinician not to assume an instructional (i.e., corrective) role. Rather, feedback should be provided as it normally would be in a conversational misunderstanding and could be something like "Oh, I thought you meant planting the grass. He's really mowing the lawn." In this way the clinician lets the client know that she or he did not accurately receive the message, but does not introduce an instructional element into the *conversational* interaction. In PACE it is important to remember that the goal is to engage in communicative interactions that resemble natural conversation as closely as possible.

It has been mentioned previously that clinician feedback varies as a function of familiarity with an aphasic person. Such familiarity may also introduce a potentially negative variable in clinician receiver behavior. Specifically, clinicians very familiar with a particular client may at times comprehend idosyncratic symbolic forms that a less familiar receiver may not be likely to understand. It is important that a clinician refrain from indicating such comprehension, because the overall goal of PACE in particular (and aphasia treatment in general) is to assist an aphasic person in the development of generalizable communicative behavior. Thus, in order to ensure provision of feedback that is truly relative to message adequacy, the clinician should maintain objectivity. We recommend the periodic use of a less familiar receiver in the treatment interaction in order to maximize receiver objectivity on the part of the clinician. A clinician can then observe such an interaction and compare his or her typical feedback responses with that of the less familiar receiver. Also, this strategy provides practice with respect to one type of extralinguistic context, namely, people.

As a final comment, we want to mention that clinicians may frequently encounter aphasic persons who are not satisfied with sending an adequate message. Such persons usually feel it is more important to verbalize perfectly and are not satisfied with successful communication per se. We want to stress that in PACE it is of the utmost importance for the clinician to initially provide feedback based on communicative adequacy. A clinician may then additionally comment by verbally affirming the client's message. Many clients may then choose to repeat such affirmations. Such an activity on the part of a client would be incidental to the PACE interaction, but it may relieve some clients' frustration with respect to need for verbalization.

Unfortunately, many aphasic persons will never verbalize as well as they would like, and continued attempts to verbalize beyond their means may be frustrating and self-defeating (Wilcox and Davis, 1977). As Holland (1978) has pointed out, the clinician, aphasic person, and family members must face the reality of residual verbal limitations. This requires a clinician to counsel a client and his or her family regarding the adequacy and use of communicative channels. Sometimes, in order to facilitate family members' acceptance of a variety of communicative channels, it may be useful to conduct a PACE interaction with a client and his or her family members.

ADJUSTING PACE TO MEET INDIVIDUAL NEEDS

PACE can be designed for aphasic clients presenting all types and levels of impairment. The basic reason for this flexibility is our assumption that any aphasic individual can communicate basic ideas in some way. The purpose of this section is to more fully detail the various ways in which PACE can be individualized. Due to the emphasis on message adequacy some clinicians may view PACE as a procedure to be used when a client is not capable of verbal activity. Conversely, some clinicians may view PACE as being too high level for low-functioning aphasic persons. Neither of these views represents an accurate concept of PACE. In our clinical experience we have successfully used PACE with a wide variety of aphasic persons (see case studies presented in Chapter 6). Such success has been achieved by selecting conversational stimuli, communicative channels, sending criteria, and modeling in accordance with a particular client's interests and level of functioning. Table 4-2 summarizes the relevant parameters of these areas of adjustment.

In order to make appropriate adaptations in PACE it is important that a clinician understand a client's communicative functioning. Hence it is necessary to have conducted a thorough pragmatic analysis of an

Table 4-2.   Areas of Adjustment for a PACE Activity

Conversational Stimuli
  Topic (e.g., occupations, family members)
  Manner of symbolic representation (e.g., pictures, photographs, written material)
  Type of message represented (e.g., abstract versus concrete, single versus multiple concepts)

Sending and Receiving Criteria
  One concept (e.g., noun or object name)
  Multiple concepts (e.g., actor + action + object, or multiple sentences)

Communicative Channels
  Speech
  Gesture
    Pointing (to pictures, words, letters, objects)
    Symbolic (e.g., illustrating functions, or more formal gestural systems such as Amer-Ind)
  Writing
  Drawing

Clinician Modeling
  Channel selection
  Communicative and linguistic complexity

---

aphasic person's communicative interactions (see Chapter 3). This sort of information (e.g., successful and unsuccessful communicative strategies, specific interests, nature of previous or ongoing work experiences) will serve as the basis for making adaptations with the PACE procedure.

Conversational Stimuli

Initially, a clinician needs to consider the stimuli that serve as topics for conveying messages. There are three basic considerations with respect to stimulus selection. These include the general topic, the symbolic representation of the stimuli, and the type of message that is represented. The message stimuli should consist of topics that are of interest to a client. Potential topics may be those corresponding to a client's work, family, hobby, or any preferred activity. Examples of considerations with respect to topic selection can be found in case studies presented in Chapter 6.

Once general topic areas have been identified, considerations should be given with respect to the manner in which the topics are represented on stimulus cards. Options include pictures (either actual or drawn), written material, or a combination of pictures and written material. In terms of difficulty, written material may prove the most challenging for most aphasic persons. Thus, we generally recommend that pictures be employed with lower functioning clients and written language with higher functioning clients.

Following selection of a symbolic format, there are several options for the type of message that is to be represented. Initially, clinicians should decide whether message types represent single or multiple concepts. Within each of these categories, further options include objects, persons, or actions whose representations may vary along a continuum of abstractness. Thus, some message types may be represented as stimuli for which communication can be accomplished with a single word or gesture, and other message types may require a larger or more complex amount of communicative behavior in order to be transmitted effectively.

The degree of difficulty a patient may experience with a particular message type will vary not only according to the level of aphasic impairment but also in accordance with the type of aphasic syndrome. For example, it may seem intuitively obvious that a pictured concrete object may represent one of the easier types of message stimuli, since communication can be accomplished with a single word or gesture. For aphasic clients exhibiting word retrieval difficulties accompanied by circumlocutionary behaviors, such stimuli may prove to be very difficult. With such clients, stimuli with more than one concept (e.g., a barnyard scene) offer a wider choice of ideas to convey on any one turn. Thus, our recommendation for selection of message types to keep in mind is that message types vary in terms of communicative difficulty. Further, such variance cannot be described in general parameters and is best approached on an individualized basis with each aphasic client.

Sending and Receiving Criteria

Another parameter to consider in the adjustment of PACE is the sending and receiving criteria for a given client. We have typically defined such criteria in terms of number of concepts that must be sent or received. In general, fewer concepts would be associated with lower functioning clients, and a larger number of concepts with higher functioning clients (unless, for example, having a choice among a larger number of concepts is easier for a particular client).

The specific concept criterion may influence the selection of message types discussed in the previous section. For example, if a clinician is requiring three concepts to be conveyed about each topic, there are two ways in which this can be accomplished. One method would involve a message type that represents a single item (e.g., a golf club). In order to specify the communication of three concepts with this type of message the clinician would initiate the PACE activity by informing the client that they were going to take turns letting each other know three things about each of the topics. The specifics of those three concepts would be up to the sender, since the message stimuli only specify the general topic.

A second method for eliciting three concepts per topic could be accomplished by adjusting the message types such that on each stimulus card three specific concepts are represented. The instruction at the initiation of a PACE activity with these forms of messages would be something like "We're going to take turns letting each other know everything that is on the cards." In this second method, the information to be conveyed is not left up to the sender, rather, it is clearly depicted on the message stimuli. However, the channels and lexical-syntactic forms used to convey these concepts are still a matter of choice for the client. In comparing this technique with the first one described (i.e., patient generates information), it is difficult to say which might be more difficult. As with message types, difficulty may vary as a function of level, as well as type, of aphasia. It would seem that the method in which three distinct concepts are represented on a stimulus card might be a more concrete communicative task and, therefore, easier for some clients.

Communicative Channels

A third area to consider in the process of adjusting PACE relates to the communicative channels that are made available or emphasized with an aphasic client. A clinician should have initial impressions relative to appropriate communicative channels that are based upon formal assessments. It is likely that such impressions are either negated or reinforced through more informal pragmatically oriented assessment. Following such assessment, a clinician will probably have a relatively accurate idea as to optimal communicative channels with which to begin the treatment process. For example, a formal test may reveal that a particular client has relatively limited verbal functioning but seems less impaired in terms of writing. More informal testing might reveal that the client occasionally relies on writing letters or parts of words in order to convey a message. With such a client, an initial channel to be made available would probably be writing. Or, a client might be observed, on occasion, to write in the air with a finger. The use of a channel such as this should be encouraged in a PACE interaction.

In selecting communicative channels a clinician needs to be careful. Specifically, he or she should ensure that the aphasic person experiences a reasonable degree of success in communicating. Thus, the initial channels emphasized should be those that have been identified as successful communicative strategies for the client. Over time it is likely that clients' optimal communicative channels will change, and such changes may be the result of directed (traditional) treatment exercises. The clinician should be sensitive to such changes in needs (and desires) and provide expanded versions of old channels or entirely new channels.

Clinicians should also be aware of the fact that messages can frequently be conveyed effectively with channel combinations and, therefore, should encourage the use of such combinations. Frequently a treatment starting point may be with channel combinations. For example, a client with limited verbal abilities and relatively good gestural skills should be provided with opportunities and encouragement to use combinations of these channels. By themselves, each channel may be ineffective, but used together, they may provide the right combination of cues to convey a message. We encourage gestures alone only as a "last resort," when all efforts to facilitate verbalization have met with little success. Generally, encouragement of channel use is provided through modeling, an adjustment process that is discussed in the next section.

Clinician Modeling

The fourth and potentially most crucial area of adjustment for PACE concerns clinician modeling, both in the sending and receiving roles. It is through these roles that aphasic persons have the opportunity to observe natural use of their optimal communicative channels. We recommend that clinicians initiate the PACE process by modeling a variety of channels that have been selected as desirable for a given client. Then, through observations of a client's preferences, the clinician should focus on refining use of those particular channels.

The preceding recommendation does not mean that clinicians should only model channels that are preferred by a client. Modeling of nonpreferred channels would be appropriate if a client's use of the channels would be likely to result in improved communication. For example, an aphasic client may experience general success with gestures, but he or she may also have some degree of potential with speech. Because there are times when gestures can be difficult to interpret, a clinician may want to model the use of gestures in combination with speech or, occasionally, the use of speech in isolation.

Clinicians may also choose to model nonpreferred channels in instances in which a client is relying too heavily on a channel that may not always be available. For example, let us consider a client whose written language recognition abilities are relatively good. This client may use a notebook, as a means of expression, that contains various important words and phrases. In the event that this client should ever be found without her notebook, alternative communicative or backup communicative strategies should become a part of the PACE interaction in the form of clinician modeling. Also, sometimes clients' preferences with respect to communicative channels may not be realistic. For example, a client with very limited verbal abilities may frequently attempt, unsuccessfully, to verbalize messages. In cases such as these, clinicians should model use of potentially successful alternative communicative strategies.

Adjustments: Final Comments

In general we have found that PACE can be successfully adjusted so that most clients can experience successful communication. We therefore believe that many aphasic clients can benefit from treatment that includes a PACE interaction. We do not mean to suggest that PACE should comprise the sole or entire treatment focus. In fact, there is probably no one single treatment procedure that could presume to be effective in isolation for all types and levels of aphasic impairment. Further, there are a number of other methods, in addition to PACE, that can be used to incorporate pragmatic variables into the treatment process.

As noted several times previously, in PACE clinicians do not directly instruct clients in the use of communicative strategies or message types. Rather, clinicians model the use of optimal communicative strategies. In the process of such modeling, clinicians may find, even though they are modeling certain strategies or channels frequently, that clients are still not incorporating certain channels or strategies in the PACE interaction. In cases such as these, a clinician should probably terminate the PACE interaction and focus on specific and direct channel stimulation or instruction. This is not to say that we would recommend abandonment of PACE. Rather, we would recommend that PACE interactions serve as the opportunity for clients to "try out" channels that have been the focus of direct instruction.

OBSERVING COMMUNICATIVE CHANGE IN PACE

The unique nature of PACE does not make it amenable to traditional methods of scoring a client's communicative successes. Specifically, scoring systems based upon correct or incorrect responses are not totally appropriate, because the primary response requirement in PACE is for a client to adequately communicate messages that are initially unknown to clinicians. Further, in order to plan clinician behavior in a PACE interaction, some knowledge of a client's communicative effectiveness and its relationship to channel use is necessary. Thus clinical observations of communicative behavior in PACE should have a focus on communicative effectiveness and specific channel use.

A method we have found useful for documenting communicative effectiveness involves determining a client's effectiveness for each message sent. In order to accomplish this, we have typically employed a rating scale. We discussed rating scales for conversation in Chapter 3, and many of those techniques could also be appropriate for rating a PACE interaction. At this time we want to consider two rating methods that were specifically designed for PACE and are both based generally upon the number of mini-turns that occur before a clinician accurately comprehends a message.

One scale, which was developed by Davis (1980) appears in Table 4-3. This scale assigns numerical values to clients' success in communicating a message when they are serving as a topic initiator or sender. Thus this scale focuses upon the more global turn-taking level that was discussed in the *Equal Participation* section of this chapter. Global turns begin when a client selects a stimulus card and terminate when it becomes a clinician's turn to select a card. As can be seen upon examining the scale, communicative success depends upon the type as well as amount of feedback that is provided by a clinician.

We shall consider several examples as a means of illustrating use of the scale display in Table 4-3. Our first example includes the following sequence:

Client: (selects picture) "eat" (brings hand from surface of table to mouth repeatedly)
Clinician: "I understand. Someone is eating."
Client: "That's right."

In this example a rating of 5 would be assigned. The message was conveyed on the client's first attempt. A rating of 4 would be assigned if the next sequence occurred:

Client: (selects picture) "Face" (holds hand flat along jaw)
Clinician: (imitates gesture) "Something about your face?"
Client: "Yes, on face." (makes shaving motion)
Clinician: "Oh, I get it. Shaving. You mean shaving."
Client: "That's right."

In this second example a rating of 4 is assigned since the clinician provided feedback, in a questioning manner, indicating the message was not understood. The client was able to successfully repair the message by including additional gestural information.

Our next example illustrates a turn that would be assigned a rating of 3.

Client: (selects picture) ". . . fire."
Clinician: "A fire?"
Client: "No. It's a. . . a. . . fire."
Clinician: "I'm not sure, something is burning? Is there anything else you can let me know?"
Client: (gestures bringing two fingers to mouth) "smoke. . . smoking"
Clinician: "Oh, I understand. A cigarette. You're talking about a cigarette."
Client: "That's right, good."

In this third example the clinician initially provided general feedback (e.g., "fire?"). The client was still unable to convey the message so the clinician provided more specific feedback that included a guess as well as a request for additional information. The client was able to formulate a successful repair after the second round of feedback.

Our fourth example illustrates a rating of 2. The specific components include provision of general and specific feedback by the clinician. In this example the client is never able to formulate an entirely successful repair, and the message is only partially conveyed. Ratings of 2 are assigned when messages are partially conveyed *only* after general and specific feedback has been attempted.

> Client: (selects picture) "Uh. . . floor. . . wall. . . yeah." (waves hand back and forth)
> Clinician: "Something about floor or wall?" (imitates gesture)
> Client: "Yeah, floor." (draws a square)
> Clinician: "Something about the floor. It's square." (points to square drawn by client) "A tile?"
> Client: "Yes, the floor." (points to square)
> Clinician: "I don't quite get it. The floor tile?
> Client: "Yes, see." (shows picture in which a person is putting tiles on a bathroom wall)

A rating of 1 would be assigned if a patient conveys information that is not related or appropriate to the topic, despite a clinician's provision of general and specific feedback. If, for example, in the preceding sequence the client had had a picture of someone hanging a painting, then the communicative attempt would have been assigned a score of 1. Ratings of 0 are reserved for those instances in which a client makes no attempt to communicate a message as in the following:

> Client: (selects picture) "uh. . . no. . . I can't."
> Clinician: "You can't let me know?"
> Client: "No, I don't know."
> Clinician: "Is there anything you can let me know?"
> Client: "No."
> Clinician: "Okay, I'll take a turn."

Although the rating scale described by Davis (1980) is useful for evaluating many aspects of a PACE interaction, there are some sequences that it is not designed to rate. For example, consider the following sequence:

> Client: (selects picture) "Man. . . tiles. . . on floor"
> Clinician: "A man putting tiles on the floor?"
> Client: "That's right." (shows picture of someone putting tiles on a wall)

In this example, only partial information was conveyed, but the clinician provided neither general nor specific feedback; she thought she had the appropriate interpretation from the first communication. On the scale appearing in Table 4–3 a score of 2 is reserved for partial communications,

Table 4-3. Rating Scale for a PACE Interaction

Score	Definition
5	Message conveyed on first attempt. There are two definitions of best performance: (1) message is conveyed by client with combined active participation of the client's sending behavior and the clinician's ability to make an appropriate interpretation from information given by the client, acknowledging the usual contribution of the receiver in any conversation or (2) a specified required completeness of the client's sending behavior in terms of number of concepts conveyed, minimizing the clinician's filling in of missing parts and placing a greater burden on the client for the communication.
4	Message conveyed as above (either 1 or 2) after general feedback from the clinician indicating the first attempt had not been completely understood. This includes the clinician's repeating the client's attempt in a questioning fashion.
3	Message conveyed as above (either 1 or 2) after specific feedback. This feedback reflects the clinician's assuming an active role as receiver in determining the client's message, either by proposing hypotheses about the messages (topic, semantic relations) or by suggesting an additional channel be used ("Show me," "Tell me anything about it"). Clinicians sometimes risk pursuing this level of feedback too long, especially having ignored that the message was conveyed. Because of the varied types and amounts of feedback possible, this category might be differentiated into a greater number of scale points in order to make the scale more sensitive to efficiency.
2	Message partially conveyed by the client, only after general (point 4) and specific (point 3) feedback have been attempted.
1	Message not conveyed appropriately despite efforts by the patient and clinician reflected in points 4 and 3.
0	Client does not attempt to convey the message.
U	Unscorable response, usually because one or more of the principles of PACE were violated in the interaction.

From Davis, G. (1980). A critical look at PACE therapy. In R. Brookshire (Ed.), *Clinical Aphasiology Conference proceedings.* Minneapolis: BRK Publishers. Reprinted with permission.

but only after general and specific clinician feedback. Hence, future applications of the scale may need to include provisons for scoring partial success that is not dependent upon the amount or type of feedback provided by a clinician.

Another means of evaluating communicative effectiveness in PACE includes notations relative to the number of mini-turns exchanged between a clinician and client prior to message comprehension. Unlike the scale represented in Table 4-3, this method is designed to score client receiving and sending behavior. The number of turns exchanged when a client is sending a message will count as his or her sending score for that particular stimulus item. The number of turns exchanged when a clinician is sending a message will count as the client's receiving score for that stimulus item. An example of this type of scoring can be found in Table 4-4.

Table 4-4.   Scoring Client Turns

Score	Examples
1R	Clinician: (selects picture) "I wash my hands with this." Client: "Soap." Clinician: "That's it, soap, a bar of soap."
2S	Client: (selects picture) ". . . fire." Clinician: "Fire? . . . I'm not sure what you mean." Client: "Smoke, smoking." (gestures bringing two fingers to mouth) Clinician: "Oh, I know, smoking a cigarette." Client: "That's right, good."
2R	Clinician: (selects picture) "A man is reading a newspaper." Client: "Huh?" Clinician: "Newspaper." (gestures turning of pages) Client: "Oh, okay." (points to picture of newspaper) Clinician: "Yea, that's what I mean."

R = Receiver turn; S = Sender turn.

Finally, it should be mentioned that both of the scoring methods we have described evaluate *overall* communicative effectiveness. Neither method includes specific provisions for evaluation of specific communicative strategies, that is, particular channels used for communication. It is also important to record specific channels being used by a patient and the degree of success associated with the channels being used. This assessment can be easily accomplished with both of the scoring methods we have discussed. In assigning ratings, or turn scores, a clinician simply needs to note the specific channel being used. In this way an inventory is generated whereby channel use can be correlated with communicative effectiveness.

Regardless of the scoring format being applied, it is initially necessary to obtain an appropriate sample of PACE interaction. Our clinical observation has been that 30 global turns (i.e., patient is sender or initiator 15 times and receiver 15 times) usually yields representative information for a probe that is conducted approximately every fourth treatment session. Of course, a clinician may alternatively choose to score turns from every treatment session. Samples can be scored from videotapes or a live observation. We have generally found that videotapes are easier because one is less likely to miss important aspects of patient behavior. Scoring during an actual treatment session is not easy because a clinician must alternate attention between modeling appropriate sending and receiving behavior *and* evaluating a behavior. However, this form of live observation is more feasible if a second clinician is available for scoring. Of the two specific methods we have discussed, the one scoring the number of turns (Table 4-4) is easier to use for a live observation.

Thus far we have discussed observation of communicative change at a rather general level. Frequently in PACE a clinician may be interested in different patient behavior during different points in treatment. For example, an initial goal may be to increase a patient's use of contingent queries. Evaluation would therefore be focused upon documenting specific changes in the use of such queries. Or, a clinician may be interested in increasing a patient's use of a particular communicative channel such as gestures. In this case the primary evaluatory focus would be upon use of gestures. The point is that a clinician will certainly want to periodically evaluate overall communicative effectiveness and correlate it with channel use. However, the day-to-day treatment data may include more specific measures of communicative behavior.

EFFICACY OF PACE

Our clinical observations, as well as pre- and post-treatment and ongoing treatment comparisons, have indicated that PACE is an effective treatment procedure in terms of improving aspects of clients' communicative abilities. However, we recognize the need to address the efficacy issue from a carefully planned research perspective. Although our formal research with PACE has not been extensive, to date we have completed two investigations of the PACE procedure. One investigation employed a repeated-measures group design, and the other was in the form of a single-case design.

Group Investigation

We shall first consider the group investigation. This study was designed to compare the effects of PACE versus direct stimulation of impaired modalities on the communicative and symbolic abilities of aphasic clients. The treatment sessions involving direct stimulation consisted of situations in which the clinician instructed the client to communicate about stimulus items with a particular communicative channel while also providing corrective feedback and cuing techniques in attempts to maximize symbolic accuracy.

In the study a total of eight aphasic persons served as participants. The clients ranged in age from 33 to 61 years with a mean age of 50. The years post onset for the clients ranged from 1 to 10 with a mean of 3.3. The types of aphasic impairment included Wernicke's (1), Broca's (5), anomic (1), and global (1). All clients had been receiving some form of treatment (either individual or group) since the onset of aphasic impairment.

At the initiation of the study all clients were given two pretest measures. These included the *Porch Index of Communicative Ability* (PICA) (Porch, 1967) and a role-playing battery. The role-playing battery was similar to role-playing techniques described in Chapter 3 and included a total of 12 common situations (e.g., finding something in a store, locating a doctor's office) that the client was asked to act out with the tester. Client communicative behaviors were scored as a function of the number of predetermined prompts (up to a maximum of three) that needed to be supplied by the tester in order for a message to be conveyed. The best score that could be obtained for a given situation was four; one point was subtracted for each prompt that had to be supplied by a tester. Scores were then summed and converted to percentages by dividing the number of points gained by the client (e.g., 46) by the number of points possible (48) and multiplying by 100.

These testing procedures were repeated either one or two times during the investigation. All testing was conducted by the same individual. Twenty-five per cent of the PICA's and 25 per cent of the role-playing tests were videotaped for purposes of scoring by an independent observer. Computation of percentage of agreement revealed reliability levels of 96 per cent for the PICA and 91 per cent for the role-playing batteries.

Following pretesting the clients were randomly assigned to one of two experimental groups. One group received PACE treatment for four weeks, at a rate of two individual sessions per week, and the other group continued to receive the treatment described as directed stimulation of impaired communicative modalities, also at a rate of two individual sessions per week. A different clinician conducted treatment for each participant group. At the end of the four week period all clients were again given the tests described in the previous paragraph. Following this, the group who had been receiving directed treatment was exposed to four weeks of PACE, again at a rate of two individual sessions per week. At the end of this second four week period, testing was again conducted.

Two general comparisons were of interest in the investigation. The first comparison was made between the two groups of clients at the end of the first four week phase. At this point we examined the effects of PACE versus direct stimulation treatment. The second comparison was made within the clients and focused on changes made during the phases of the study in which they were exposed to PACE. The comparison of PACE with direct stimulation treatment was accomplished by computing difference scores for each client from their initial pretests to the repeated tests at the end of the first four week phase. Separate analyses were performed for the role-playing battery, the overall PICA scores and PICA verbal scores. The specific data for each of these analyses can be found in Tables 4-5, 4-6, and 4-7. For each set of data, a Mann Whitney U Test was performed. Results indicated that those clients exposed to PACE performed significantly better (p < .05) on the role-playing measure and the PICA verbal scores. No differences were apparent between the two groups with respect to overall PICA scores. Comparison of the overall effects of PACE for all of the clients was accomplished by performing a Wilcoxon Matched Pairs Test for the same three parameters described previously. These data can also be seen in Tables 4-5, 4-6, and 4-7. Results indicated significant change (p < .05) in performance on the role-playing battery and the PICA verbal subtests during the PACE phases of the study.

Single Case Study

In this investigation, a 55 year old woman with global aphasia served as the participant. She was six months post onset at the time of the investigation and had been receiving treatment for approximately two months. The design was in the form of an ABCBC time series format. The treatment phases of the investigation (BCBC) included PACE (B) and direct stimulation of impaired modalities (C), with the direct stimulation being in the same format as was described for the group investigation. Each treatment phase consisted of eight sessions that occurred at a rate of four times per week.

Two baseline measures were initially taken. These were followed by 32 treatment sessions in which the two different procedures were alternated every eight sessions. Thus there were two PACE phases and two direct stimulation phases. The same clinician conducted all treatment sessions. During the treatment phases, probe measures were taken after every two sessions. All measures (baseline and probes) were in the form of a role-playing battery. The same role-playing battery and scoring procedures that were used for the group investigation were applied here.

The results of the role-playing measures for each phase of the study can be seen in Figure 4-1. Upon examining the figure, an approximation of a stairstep effect can be seen. In general, the larger amount of improvement is associated with the PACE phases of the study.

Summary of Research

As mentioned previously, the research we have conducted thus far is not extensive. However, the results of even these limited investigations can be viewed as promising. In both investigations patients made improvement during the PACE phases that was not observed during

Table 4-5. Role-Playing Scores (per cent)

Group A	Pre	PACE	Post		
	69	+ 22	91		
	82	+ 10	92		
	57	+ 20	77		
	75	+ 13	88		
Group B	Pre	DS	Pre 2	PACE	Post
	76	+ 1	77*	—	—
	49	+ 9	58	+ 20	78
	52	+ 7	59	+ 25	84
	65	+ 1	66	+ 13	79

DS = Direct stimulation of impaired channels.
*This client moved before the second phase of the study was completed.

Table 4-6. Pre-Post PICA Verbal Percentile Scores

Group A	Pre	PACE	Post		
	78	+ 4	82		
	71	+ 3	74		
	51	+ 1	52		
	75	0	75		
Group B	Pre	DS	Pre 2	PACE	Post
	75	− 6	69*	—	—
	50	0	50	+ 7	57
	48	− 1	47	+ 4	51
	53	− 2	51	+ 1	52

DS = Direct stimulation of impaired channels.
*This client moved before the second phase of the study was completed.

Table 4-7. Pre-Post PICA Overall Percentile Scores

Group A	Pre	PACE	Post		
	83	− 3	82		
	83	+ 1	84		
	65	− 1	64		
	76	+ 8	84		
Group B	Pre	DS	Pre 2	PACE	Post
	91	+ 4	95*	—	—
	53	+ 5	58	+ 4	65
	45	+ 3	40	+ 4	52
	72	− 8	64	+ 5	69

DS = Direct stimulation of impaired channels.
*This client moved before the second phase of the study was completed.

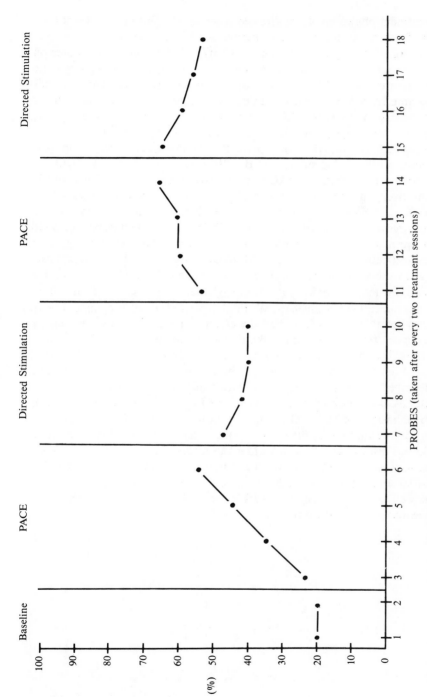

Figure 4–1. Comparison of PACE and directed stimulation.

treatment phases involving directed stimulation. This improvement took the form of an increase in communicative effectiveness with the role-playing situations and, for some patients, an increase in their scores on the verbal subtests of the PICA. The role-playing battery was pragmatic in nature, as is PACE. Therefore, changes in performance on this parameter, relative to the more directed treatment, were not particularly surprising. That is, in PACE the focus is on communicative adequacy. In the role-playing measures the focus was also on communicative adequacy. The fact that some patients demonstrated an increase in their scores on the verbal subtests of the PICA was unexpected. We had not expected the effects of PACE to be associated with specific linguistic improvement that was not pragmatic in nature. Wilcox and Davis (1977) made a suggestion that offers an explanation for this unexpected improvement in some of our patients. They believe that when patients were not primarily concerned with linguistic perfection they were actually more linguistically adequate. They additionally suggested that many aphasic patients may focus too heavily on producing linguistically acceptable communicative behavior, thereby inadvertently limiting their communicative effectiveness. We think it possible that the communicative focus of PACE may have had the effect, for some patients, of causing them to "think" less about talking and, as was suggested by Wilcox and Davis, become more linguistically adequate in the process.

Finally, we want to remind the reader that the studies we have described were not designed to assess treatment effectiveness per se. Rather they assessed the relative effectiveness of PACE versus another approach to aphasia treatment. Overall, it appears that PACE is a treatment procedure that is capable of improving aphasic persons' communicative skills. Future research, with a wider variety and larger number of aphasic persons would seem to be warranted in order to further substantiate this initial conclusion. It is our hope that our detailed descriptions of PACE, as well as other pragmatic variables related to aphasia treatment, will encourage such future research.

Chapter 5

Treatment in the Pragmatic Domain

Having presented a procedure that models the structure of conversation, we now extend our discussion of treatment into all areas of pragmatics as outlined in Chapter 1. We have shown how contextual variables comprise a substantial portion of communication and, of particular relevance for aphasia, how these variables influence the language behavior of normal and aphasic adults. With Chapter 4 as a springboard, we are demonstrating the third and fourth steps in the development of treatment strategies, namely, presenting ideas concerning relevant treatment procedures and reporting on how most of these have been conducted with aphasic patients.

This chapter has two major orientations. The primary orientation is aimed at improvement of an aphasic patient's communicative behaviors. The other is directed at improving the patient's communicative contexts. As we deal with improving the patient, we shall be presenting suggestions for the treatment of verbal and nonverbal communicative behavior and for the incorporation of internal and external contexts in this treatment.

RATIONALE

Since the treatment of aphasia on a wide scale began in the 1940s, clinicians have yearned for ways to develop systems that could be used conveniently in a clinic and that also would reflect the use of language outside of the clinic. The extensive practice of "naming" seemed to be valid because at least it is one form of word retrieval, the heart of an aphasic person's expressive difficulty. Yet, confrontation naming seemed to be awkward, because people do not go around naming things too often when they leave the clinic. As another example, training the production of "want juice," "want coffee," and so on was consistent with systematic paradigms arising from behavior modification technologies, and it appeared to be relevant, because adults drink juice and coffee. However, such targets can be questioned as to their naturalness, because people do not talk with such stiff forms and do not often want or need to talk about "wanting coffee" except when meal service is not at the moment being offered in a hospital. Pragmatics, as it is developing at this moment, is giving definition to variables that influence how people talk and what people talk about. With this definition, clinicians are collecting ideas as to how components of natural linguistic performance can be managed in a clinic.

Modern pragmatics has been readily accepted by clinicians who already have expressed a need to be realistic and natural in their treatment of aphasia. A major focus has been on assisting the patient in improving what is the basic objective of language behavior, namely, communication. As a result, it has appeared that pragmatic treatment consists mainly of training in augmentative or alternative modes of communication. In this historical context, Rosenbek (1983) characterized pragmatics as follows: "Some of us can be most pragmatic when we are having the least success helping the speaker. When he cannot change, we feel that we and the rest of his environment must" (p. 320). Even PACE therapy has been associated only with treatment of nonverbal behavior (e.g., Code and Muller, 1983) and has been associated with suspicions that the pragmatic clinician is turning away from treatment of language behavior. Rosenbek's statement refers to one area of pragmatic objectives, namely, the goal of improving a patient's contexts. Yet, a possibly more important area of pragmatic treatment is to improve a patient's verbal and nonverbal behavior with clinical application of the contexts in which these communicative modes are used. As pragmatics is defined as the relationships between language behavior and contexts, pragmatic treatment is treatment of language behavior.

Pragmatic treatment is consistent with traditional stimulation and behavior modification methodologies. In fact, we do not suggest that it is necessarily a different approach that should be "added" to these more traditional ones. In this regard, we agree with Spradlin and Siegel's (1982) critique of behavior modification in the treatment of children. They argued that this procedure can be done with stimuli that are natural with respect to a client's real world and with responses that are consistent with how a client is most likely to talk outside of the clinic. In making these suggestions, Spradlin and Siegel were addressing the basic clinical problem of *generalization* of gains seen in treatment activity to the use of treated behaviors outside of the clinic. They suggested that generalization is most likely to occur when treatment is most reflective of natural language contexts and behavior. We suggest that the domain of pragmatics assists the clinician in identifying components of natural language behavior that can be inserted into a clinical program of rehabilitation. In applying these components, a clinician may conduct stimulation or behavior modification or both pragmatically.

There are some general principles by which direct treatment can be constructed so that it represents characteristics of natural communicative contexts:

1. Natural use of language presents the individual with a *variety* of communication problems. Real life does not present one form of discourse structure, only neutral emotions, one purpose, one other conversational participant, one degree of shared knowledge, and so on. Along with variety comes the unexpected, and anxiety may come from the unexpected. People differ from each other with respect to the variety of situations they are willing to confront. Additional restrictions in the willingness to participate in different contexts may result from an aphasic person's psychological response to his or her disability, as well as the disability itself. Therefore, the variety of treatment contexts should be realistic relative to the individual aphasic person's likely possibilities outside of the clinic.

2. Natural use of language often involves some *miscommunication*. Aphasic persons, in particular, will make mistakes and fail to retrieve sufficient language outside of the clinic. Yet, in a well-constructed session of traditional language drill, a client may experience success most of the time (e.g., Brookshire, 1978; Davis, 1983). The rationale behind providing conditions for consistent success is certainly valid, because practice with a language process can only be achieved when it is resulting in success and is free from the frustration of error. However, a client is not exposed to such carefully designed situations in natural contexts. We hope that success in drill results in improvement of language processing that is sufficient to overcome natural obstacles, but the ability to deal with error should also be a concern during a session of treatment.

LINGUISTIC CONTEXT

In the 1960s, treatment centered on the word as the basic unit of controlled stimulation. In the 1970s, clinicians became more systematic in the manipulation of sentence-level variables. Now, clinicians may deal with the intersentential level of language with a heightened sensitivity as to its unique structural features. The structure of discourse and text can be used to define variables of stimulation and parameters of expected response within the four major modalities of language behavior.

Comprehension

Objectives for improving comprehension might include targeting areas of difficulty in processing microstructural coherence devices. This relatively untried realm of treatment has few procedural models to follow from basic research. The targets consist of referential coherence devices such as pronouns and articles. The most appropriate patient would be one with mild comprehension impairment. Patients may practice identifying the antecedents of pronominal and article designations of given information. At the intersentential level, these antecedents should occur in a previous sentence that is paired with a sentence containing a pronoun or article (see examples in Chapters 1 and 2). One treatment manual contains auditory problems such as the following (Martinoff, Martinoff, and Stokke, 1980, p. 153): "A jet plane flew over my house last night. It made a lot of noise. What made a lot of noise?" Answering the question implies that the listener should know the antecedent for "it." However, in the manual, not all items of the task are focused on making such an intersentential connection. In fact, in some items, the second sentence is not necessary at all for answering a question. It appears that awareness of microstructural devices can contribute a sharper focus on the kinds of language processes being practiced in a multisentential drill.

Processing difficulty is raised when the distance between given information and the first mention of it is increased. Furthermore, auditory presentation would reasonably consist of sentence pairs, with a printed version as simultaneous support or as a cue in response to the occurrence of error. The printed version could be presented for a response that entails pointing to the antecedent. With reading as the focus of attention, visual presentation may involve less concern with short-term memory demands and, therefore, may consist of longer paragraphs.

A common activity involving practice at the intersentential level is a reading task in which printed sentences are arranged in an order that is consistent with appropriate text structure. At the microstructural level, sentences can be prepared so that new information is in one sentence, and coreference devices referring back to new information are in other sentences. At the macrostructural level, one variable in such a task would include different types of text, such as narrative and procedural formats.

The macrostructural level of standard activity consists of presenting paragraphs to either receptive modality. This level is usually reserved for mild comprehension impairment, and clinicians draw from newspaper articles and clients' favorite reading materials for auditory or visual content. Mildly impaired patients usually possess enough verbal expression so that controlling for simplicity of response is not as important as it is for patients whose verbal output is an effort or is incomprehensible.

Patients may be asked to (a) summarize or paraphrase what was heard or read, (b) tell the main point or theme, or (c) answer specific questions about the content of a paragraph. With respect to answering questions, these may be designed to ask about main points, details, explicit information, or implicit information (e.g., Brookshire and Nicholas, 1984). In fact, through these methods, a patient can be focused on problems sometimes found in mild aphasias, as Butler wrote in describing his comprehension difficulties: ". . . difficulties in conversation arise mainly from my seemingly frequent inability to understand adequately the main point of a discussion or the implication of a remark" (Sies and Butler, 1963, p. 265).

Published treatment materials indicate that there has been some sensitivity to variety of macrostructural form, as well as varied levels in terms of number of sentences. For example, Martinoff and coworkers (1980) provide a large number of paragraphs, some of which are narratives (i.e., stories with a sequence of events) and some of which are descriptions of people with a list of their characteristics. In addition to narration and description, the forms of discourse include exposition (i.e., explanation of a subject) and argumentation (i.e., an attempt to "prove" something with rules of logic or science) (Weaver, 1967). Procedural discourse can be added to this list.

Expression

While it seems that the discourse level of production should be practiced only by mildly impaired patients, preservation of discourse structure has been achieved by moderately impaired individuals in spite of deficiencies in word retrieval and sentence completeness. Many aphasic persons retain the capacity to tell stories with a beginning, middle, and end. In studies of *narrative* discourse production (Ulatowska, Freedman-Stern, Doyel, Macaluso-Haynes, and North, 1983), aphasic subjects achieved scores that ranged from 52 per cent (139.5 of 267) to 96 per cent (257 out of 267) on the *Boston Diagnostic Aphasia Examination* (Goodglass and Kaplan, 1972). Such patients may be presented the opportunity to practice producing the essentials of discourse with tasks such as those used by Ulatowska in her research. We suggest a hierarchy of these tasks, along with our own additions, as shown in Table 5-1. Response expectations should not be addressed to intrasentential linguistic elements, but expectations should focus the patient on preserving superstructural characteristics such as the setting, action, and resolution of a story.

The other forms of discourse should be practiced, and these include

Table 5-1.   Tasks for Eliciting Narrative Discourse*

1. Tell a story with the help of story sequence picture cards.
    a. With all cards present.
    b. From memory, after clinician removes some or all of the cards.
2. Retell a story presented by clinician, such as a familiar or unfamiliar fable.
3. A self-generated account of a memorable experience.
4. Conversation concerning an event or memorable experience.

*Ranked in order of difficulty based on nature of input, demands on recall, and data from a study by Ulatowska, Freedman-Stern, Doyel, Macaluso-Haynes, and North, (1983).

the frequently investigated *procedural* discourse (e.g., Ulatowska, Doyel, Stern, Haynes, and North, 1983). Procedural discourse consists of explanation and description of steps in carrying out a task. The hierarchy of Table 5-1 can be preserved, especially because many published picture sequences represent this form of discourse (e.g., Developmental Learning Materials, Modern Education Corporation). Examples of procedural discourse topics include changing a lightbulb, making a sandwich, shopping in a grocery store, changing a flat tire, taking a bath, and so on (see Keith, 1972). Pictured sequences can be used as part of the initial stimulus (i.e., "Tell me what this person is doing") or as a back up cue to facilitate response in a task that asks a patient simply to explain a particular procedure. Discourse elements to expect in a response include essential steps, target steps (i.e., completion of task), and optional steps that provide detail.

PARALINGUISTIC CONTEXT

Few manuals of aphasia treatment contain a section on the treatment of paralinguistic context. One reason for this is that, in spite of measured deficiencies in more severely impaired patients, impaired recognition and expression of prosody has not appeared as a significant threat to communicative ability. For what paralinguistic cues convey (see Chapter 1), there are usually ample supplemental contextual cues to these messages. Also some deficiencies in the recognition of semantic and syntactic prosodic cues are only beginning to be realized, and their significance for the patient is not well understood. Emotional prosody, in particular, can be considered to be an area of communicative strength for aphasic persons as receivers of information and, especially with fluent aphasia, as senders of information. Persons with right hemisphere brain damage may occasionally have a greater need for treatment of prosody deficiency.

Treatment paradigms can be borrowed from the experimental literature reviewed in Chapter 2, especially with respect to recognition of prosodic information. Regarding emotional prosody, semantically neutral sentences (e.g., "He watched the news") can be presented with varying emotional tone. The patient can identify the emotion by pointing to pictures of faces with different emotional expressions. Additional cues to conveyed emotion consist of inserting emotional semantic-verbal content into the sentences. Regarding semantic/syntactic prosody, one task might involve listening to words such as "convict" with different syllabic stress and pointing to the picture representing the word that was presented. Such a task may precede drill on expression of appropriate stress relative to the picture selected by a clinician. A patient may also practice turning statements into questions by simply changing intonation pattern.

EXTRALINGUISTIC CONTEXT

Because of the multifaceted nature of extralinguistic context, it can be utilized in treatment in numerous ways. Also, with the interactive nature of contextual components that was mentioned in our first chapter, in some instances the manipulation of one variable will be accompanied by changes in other variables. In this section, we shall point out how these contexts can be exploited in direct stimulation drill. We start the section with some of the planning that is needed to take full advantage of each patient's unique contexts.

Preparation

The planning of semantic content and activities of treatment includes investigation of a patient's extralinguistic contexts, internal and external. Internal contexts consist primarily of what the patient knows about the world, and external contexts include people, settings, and purposes of language behavior that are common in the patient's environment outside of the speech-language clinic. While these contexts may become targets for change, we are considering them now as sources of information that are applied to direct treatment of the patient's language disorder. This application includes the selection of lexicon and pictures to be used in stimulation drill, behavior modification procedures, or both. Individualization of treatment content is a principle that contributes to our avoidance of lists of specific stimuli to recommend for treatment. Stimuli that are common to most people constitute only a portion of pragmatic materials created from a client's own world. As a guide to completeness, we consider all of these contexts to exist along what we call horizontal and vertical dimensions.

The *horizontal dimension* contains information that is usually obtained in a personal "history." It is a record of communicative purposes, as well as people and places, in the client's current living environment: Whom does the client talk to? Where? For what purposes? What does he or she read? How often? Does the client listen to the radio or watch television? What are favorite activities, hobbies, and television programs? What does the client want to write? Finding out about settings includes investigating home, church, work, and shopping locations. People in these settings include family, friends, clergy, colleagues, and clerks. A clinician's investigation includes determining not only whom the patient talks to now but also whom the client used to talk to before onset of aphasia, has stopped talking to, and wants to talk to again. Similar considerations apply to setting, because some of these may be avoided now because of communication barriers. Furthermore, any introduction of these sources into treatment should be preceded by a realistic assessment of current linguistic abilities. In the clinic, the patient should be exposed to contextual variables that are possible to deal with outside of the clinic, given current communicative and psychological capacities.

The *vertical dimension* has received less attention for planning treatment content and activities. It includes the patient's life history and plans for the future. A strategy for obtaining a life history was suggested by Davis and Holland (1981). This strategy involves determining dates of important milestones such as graduation from school, marriage, birth of children, job starts and changes, divorce, children leaving home, retirement, and so on. Then the occurrence of these milestones is associated with a historical "time-line," whereby a clinician obtains a sense for what was happening in the world when the milestones were reached by the client. The time-line is an abbreviated history of key news events and key figures in music, movies, and sports, all of which are found readily in an almanac. By associating the patient's milestone events with commonly known key events, the clinician is familiarized with the world as it was when the patient was going to school or raising teenagers. This investigation can be especially informative for the clinician who is much younger than the client and who may have trouble recalling coursework on recent history. Finally, if there is no source of information pertaining to future plans, the client's age is one clue to whether plans might have included further occupational advancement, additional children in the family, or a retirement strategy. While aphasia may disrupt these plans, treatment and supportive counseling may be directed toward adjusting to this disruption in a realistic fashion.

Purpose

Chapter 1 briefly introduced the manner in which purpose of communication may shape the style and content of language behavior. The purpose of a communication is related to the type of activity in which a person is involved and the subject matter in the activity. Therefore, a clinician may arrange a variety of activities on a variety of subjects with the probability that a patient will have the opportunity to use language for varied purposes as a result. Practicing conversation just to practice conversation can be limiting in this regard. Purposes that may arise naturally in different activities include instructing, motivating, ventilating feelings, and so on. At a microstructural level, purposes may be identified in terms of speech acts. Also, the practice of linguistic behavior for a particular purpose may be related to a patient's needs or desires outside of the clinic. Examples of this are mildly impaired patients who may be able to return to their occupations on a limited basis, and so they may want to practice their language skills for the purpose of directing the actions of a fellow employee or for the purpose of preparing lecture material and presenting it to a class. A patient may want to practice word retrieval in order to be able to holler at friends during a softball game.

Another arena in which purpose becomes a meaningful variable is in reading and writing activities. As Holland (1978) suggested, functional treatment of reading entails presentation of what people read from day to day: phone and address numbers, phone books, product labels, street signs, movie titles, advertisements, forms, and junk mail. Linguistic requirements become more demanding for recipes, letters, newspapers, magazines, and directions for putting together a child's birthday present. Role-playing may entail practice with an emergency situation in which looking up a phone number may be part of the activity, or it may entail ordering in a restaurant with practice in the use of menus that differ as to level of linguistic difficulty. Functional writing includes signing one's name on a form, filling out checks, creating a shopping list, taking phone messages, and composing a letter. Activities are determined with respect to the type of writing activity that a client wishes and is able to accomplish. One accomplishment of treatment can involve demonstrating to an aphasic client that he or she is able to accomplish some useful goals with writing on a limited or modified basis.

Setting

Many clinicians have attempted different strategies for creating settings that would stimulate the use of language for meaningful purposes with meaningful content. This has been fairly easy for the home health professional to accomplish. In a clinic setting, on the other hand, a range of devices have been employed from the use of props on a table to the use of living room and kitchen facilities available in an institution to the use of field trips or "on location" settings outside of an institution. Ritter (1976a) described a "modular therapy" program in which treatment activities were geared toward communication likely to occur in the patient's room, a kitchen, workshop, and cafeteria. These modules existed in the clients' nursing home. One guide to the selection of activities may be the "activities of daily living" to which occupational therapy is oriented. Such a treatment program involves interdisciplinary cooperation whereby carefully defined language stimulation can be conducted by other professionals in an institutional setting.

Components of Settings. A few aphasic patients may possess additional deficiencies in recognizing components of a setting. These deficiencies appear in the form of auditory, visual, or tactile agnosias (see Chapter 2). With respect to auditory agnosia, improvement in the recognition of familiar nonverbal sounds may contribute in a small way to the ability to relate linguistic stimuli to contextual cues. Practice would entail presentation of audio-recorded sounds with the patient pointing to pictures of the sound source. Treatment may begin with same-different judgments of different and then similar sounds; or it may begin with picture choices between two very different sound sources, proceeding to an increased number of choices and increased similarity between or among them. Procedures also would include relating sounds to words and naming the sound source.

Direct Stimulation. The individualization of content for standard comprehension and production drills is drawn from study of a patient's horizontal and vertical contexts, as mentioned earlier in this section. From horizontal contexts, this material includes photographs of people, objects, and settings in the client's world outside of the clinic. Photographs may be obtained from family albums or from loaning an instant camera to the client or a family member for pictures of the client's kitchen or favorite chair. Lexicon includes names of family members and friends, in addition to terms such as "wife," "uncle," or "neighbor." Lexicon important to the client might include names of baseball players or characters in a soap opera. People may be excited about a recent middleweight championship fight or who is sleeping with whom on a television melodrama. Vertical contexts can be provided with picture books that deal with World War II or the history of television, for example. Communication about such arousing topics might require some equalizing of shared knowledge by the clinician, who should do some homework on such topics when necessary.

Pre-stimulation as Context. In Chapter 2 we reviewed research demonstrating that language comprehension can be facilitated with a picture that is presented prior to a linguistic stimulus. The picture may represent relevant contextual information (e.g., a setting). Such "pre-stimulation" has been a component of a treatment paradigm suggested by Weigl and referred to as "deblocking" (see Davis, 1983; Greimas, Jakobson, Mayenowa, et al., 1970). The pre-stimulation phase has been thought of as a means of activating relevant fields of internal context (i.e., semantic memory), thereby facilitating access to other information in that region of lexical and conceptual knowledge. This phase may be a convenient means of providing a variety of contextual information as part of a stimulus in a language comprehension or expression task. For patients who comprehend well enough, verbal presentation of a situation as pre-stimulation for a sentence comprehension task enables the clinician to create any type of context in the imagination of a patient. Paragraphs used in metaphor comprehension tasks could be considered to be a form of pre-stimulation.

Following Instructions. Another form of setting manipulation involves the use of props in a sentence comprehension task consisting of following instructions. Following instructions has been a popular form of comprehension training, because it permits a clinician to manipulate subtle dimensions of language and to observe qualitative features of errors. Tasks in which contextual influences have been intentionally excluded include modeling treatment after the Token Test (e.g., Holland and Sonderman, 1974) and manipulation of unordinary combinations of objects (e.g., Flowers and Danforth, 1979). Some instructions involve simply pointing to such things in sequence, and others involve placing objects in peculiar juxtaposition. While it is valuable to focus on language processes by minimizing contextual influences, such activity may at least be expanded to include some pragmatic considerations.

One pragmatic consideration pertains to the manipulation of contextual influences on language comprehension in following instructions. Seron and Deloche (1981) illustrated such influences with their study involving the placement of objects in spatial relationship to each other, a study mentioned in Chapter 2. Spatial relations between objects may be congruent or incongruent with the usual relations between the objects, or they may be congruent or incongruent with physical characteristics of the objects. In Seron and Deloche's experiment, children's toys were used to represent common objects in an adult's world, such as a bed and a bathroom sink. Instructions contained the prepositions "in," "on," and "under." A task with congruent relations would contain stimuli such as "Put the shoes under the bed," and such a task would be easier than one consisting of incongruent relations such as "Put the soap under the sink."

Another pragmatic consideration brings purpose into the planning of such drill activities. For what purposes does a client follow instructions in real life? Instructions often are involved in reading tasks as in directions for putting together a barbecue set, for filing income taxes, or for baking a cake. Plausible instructions include directions for getting from one place to another or directions for taking medication. These types of instructions may be designed into the shape of a drill activity, or each type of instruction may be included in an activity designed to focus on solving one particular problem. Key planning considerations include (a) identifying instructions that a client is likely to confront and (b) molding a clinical activity that either models these instructions or contains the particular processing demands of the real-life instructions.

Participants: Internal Contexts

Internal extralinguistic context consists of conditions within the patient. These conditions include the patient's knowledge of the world (i.e., semantic memory) and his or her emotional state. Experimental manipulations of knowledge have included varying familiarity of topic in studies of normal adults and varying real world plausibility of events represented by sentences in studies of aphasia. In studies of normal and brain-damaged adults, emotional arousal has been induced with provocative pictures, lexicon, and statements.

Conceptual Knowledge. As with the external context of setting, our interest in internal context involves utilizing a patient's retained knowledge most effectively in the retraining of language behaviors. Our previous discussion of the content of direct stimulation ties directly into this component of context. What a patient knows is considered in the selection of lexicon and corresponding pictures for receptive and expressive language drills. A patient's knowledge is also considered in the selection of topics for less structured interactions such as conversation and role-playing. Aphasia treatment may revolve around spoons, chairs, trees, and cats, because shared knowledge of these "topics" is assured (as opposed to the frequently professed "functionality" of practicing comprehension and production of such words). The potential for disparate sharing of knowledge between clinician and client is increased when treatment is aimed at special knowledge that the client possesses and that is not represented in commercially available materials.

Emotional State.   Common objects situated around a client are not necessarily the things that make that client happy, excited, sad, content, or contentious. What really attracts and maintains a client's attention? What makes him or her laugh? What gets under his or her skin? Arousing events often drive a person to talk, and such events often arouse an aphasic person to talk better than he or she would when asked to describe a line drawing of a man sitting in a chair. "A man washing a car" might be arousing if it reminds a client of a recent time when he felt manipulated into washing his car when he did not want to do it. "A woman baking a cake" might be arousing if it reminds a client of a recent joyous celebration. However, a clinician need not hope to be so fortunate in achieving serendipitous arousal and can present stimuli based on previously stated guidelines for generating meaningful treatment content.

Participants: External Contexts

The communicative partner in an interaction with an aphasic client contributes certain variables that can influence the client's language behavior. These variables include the partner's contribution to shared knowledge of a topic and the partner's role in the interaction. Treatment can capture an element of natural communication by the manipulation of these variables. Adjustments in the partner's contribution to shared knowledge have been implied in previous discussions of individualization of content and use of a patient's internal context. When there is a disparity between a client's knowledge of a topic and a clinician's knowledge of that topic, then the clinician should increase his or her knowledge of the topic. In possession of this knowledge, a clinician may be able to respond to a client as if the knowledge were absent or present. As a clinician becomes increasingly familiar with a client, this variable is manipulated by having a patient do PACE or some other form of interaction with less familiar persons. Also, controlled practice, as in PACE, may be done with more familiar persons such as family members.

Having a client practice communicative skills with strangers or less familiar persons also may interact with the internal context of emotional state. Such situations may induce a condition of anxiety for which a client may become better prepared. Ritter (1976b) was able to classify interactions between clients and other persons in clients' hospital rooms based on whether the contribution of the other person appeared to be supportive (or not) or threatening (or not). He concluded that patients' language performance was better in supportive and nonthreatening circumstances than it was in the more anxiety provoking circumstances. He encouraged providing a supportive environment in treatment and changing nonsupportive or threatening people so that they might become less threatening and more supportive. While this may be part of a treatment approach, it may be unrealistic to think that a clinician can eliminate all nonsupportive and threatening situations from a patient's everyday environment or, especially, from less frequent situations to which a patient might wish to return with confidence. Role-playing may be a sufficient strategy for beginning to help a client learn to use communicative skills to their fullest when presented with uncomfortable or stressful situations.

Movement

Changing the aphasic patient's nonverbal movements has ample precedence and stems from two orientations, namely, elaboration of existing gestural ability and development of new communicative modes. Both orientations are weighted by two possible movement impairments, namely, limb apraxia and asymbolia. With respect to asymbolia, this central impairment may also entail mild-to-moderate reduction of gesture recognition in some patients. Most patients, however, retain substantial gesture recognition and some gesture expression, especially signal behaviors.

As with treatment of verbal behavior, treatment of gestural behavior builds upon what the patient already can do. As noted in Chapter 3, signal behavior includes gesticulation for regulating conversation, facial expressions of affect, and natural expressive gestures such as holding one's nose in the presence of a foul odor. Just as Helm and Barresi (1980) started with involuntary speech of severely aphasic persons, unintentional gesture can be raised to a level of intentionality. Beginning with association of gesture with pictures and printed words, a program would be similar to those used to train Amer-Ind Gestural Code (e.g., Dowden, Marshall, and Tompkins, 1981; Simmons and Zorthian, 1979; Skelly, 1979). Direct training should be supplemented with a concurrent "encourage the use of" approach involving positive reinforcement of gestures in natural communicative interactions. Schlanger and Schlanger (1970) encouraged their clients to employ retained gesturing in activities referred to as "pantomime role playing."

The use of a substantial number of pantomimic gestures is a relatively novel behavior for most adults. *American Indian gestural code* (Amer-Ind) is the most frequently reported iconic symbol system that has been presented to aphasic persons (Skelly, 1979). Many of the attempts to teach Amer-Ind have been with patients who have apraxia of speech. This gestural code has been evaluated with respect to two potential benefits: (a) as an alternative mode of communication after apparent failure to achieve functional use of speech and (b) as a means of facilitating improvements in verbalization after failure of traditional treatments. The major issue with Amer-Ind has involved *acquisition* of the system in clinical and natural settings. Part of the problem has been that clinicians sometimes do not clearly specify what is meant when they report that a client has learned the system. The obscurity involves whether learning Amer-Ind transfers from abilities displayed in clinical tasks to functional use in natural contexts. We suggest at this point that this or any other new code is truly acquired when an aphasic individual uses it effectively for conversation with family and friends.

Skelly's (1979) manual on Amer-Ind illustrates over 200 symbols and presents instructions for clinical testing and training procedures. Amer-Ind is defined as being a code and not a language. That is, it is a lexicon of hand signs without rules of grammar. Therefore, when the signs are used in a logical order, the sequence possesses a telegraphic style. The signs are considered to be natural in that they are similar to pantomime and may be expressed with some variation. The code may be superimposed easily upon an individual's own gestures, thereby, diminishing the demands of "new learning."

Amer-Ind's iconicity not only dilutes its symbolic quality but also contributes to its intelligibility to receivers who do not have special training in the code. Clinicians without previous exposure to Amer-Ind were able to guess the meaning of 80 per cent of 50 signs produced by a "patient-signaler" in one of Skelly's (1979) several studies. Twenty wives, relatives, and friends of clients were able to guess 50 to 94 per cent of signs correctly without previous exposure to the code. After viewing two hours of video instruction on Amer-Ind, this group improved to 88 to 100 per cent accuracy. These high levels of "transparency" were questioned by Daniloff, Lloyd, and Fristoe (1983) in a study of 40 professional and paraprofessional health providers who were not familiar with Amer-Ind. These subjects exhibited 42 to 50 per cent comprehension of 193 signs. Daniloff suggested that his procedure was more objective than Skelly's procedure but also noted that Amer-Ind still is significantly more transparent than American Sign Language for the deaf. Daniloff presented a complete rank ordering of transparency for the 193 signs, with 61 of them having at least 80 per cent transparency. It should be noted that the 193 signs were from Skelly's 1975 demonstration videotape and not from the somewhat modified 1979 demonstration tape.

Amer-Ind training has been given primarily to people with nonfluent aphasia plus severe apraxia of speech, as opposed to fluent types of aphasia. Skelly (1979) recommended that her complete program be given to those with intact auditory language comprehension and adequate motoric competence. Hemiplegia need not be a hindrance, because only 20 per cent of the signs required both hands. The presence of limb apraxia may be a hindrance because of the use of imitation and commands in some training steps. The program follows a traditional recognition-imitation-production sequence. Variations of the program have been tried by other clinicians (e.g., Simmons and Zorthian, 1979; Dowden et al., 1981). When this training is being used to facilitate production of speech, the client may be asked to imitate and produce verbalization in association with a gesture. However, Skelly (1979) emphasized the following: "The clinician should not press for verbalization, but wait until the patient offers verbalization spontaneously" (p. 152).

Acquisition of Amer-Ind is generally determined with respect to the number of signs used successfully at particular levels of the training program. Skelly (1979) summarized several studies that were presented at a conference in 1977. They reported the number of signs used at different training levels relative to the number of signs presented at these levels. Of 20 aphasic subjects, 14 were able to imitate all signs presented, ranging from 30 to 200 signs. Achievement at the propositional level ranged from 200 (of 200 presented) to 20 (of 65 presented). From one of several field reports in which 40 subjects were presented approximately 100 signs, imitation ranged from 30 to 112 and propositional use ranged from 8 to 41 signs.

Additional single case studies have been reported. Tonkovich and Loverso (1982) trained four clients with Broca's aphasia and apraxia of speech to produce seven verb + object combinations of Amer-Ind and other gestures. Trained production of seven combinations generalized to the production of several other combinations that were not trained. However, production was measured as a response to being given the verbal form of the combination, and spontaneous use for communication was not measured. Two of these clients were reported to have been using gestures at home. In another study, a patient with Wernicke's aphasia learned to answer questions with Amer-Ind after several months of training (Simmons and Zorthian, 1979). This subject's family reported that spontaneous use occurred at home.

While Skelly (1979) has reported cases in which verbalization improved after initiation of Amer-Ind training, a few other cases have been reported in which such facilitation did not occur (Dowden et al., 1981; Simmons and Zorthian, 1979; Skelly, 1979). Rao and Horner (1978) described a program for a patient with severe aphasia in which Amer-Ind training promoted improved communicative use of gesture and improved linguistic performance on formal tasks. With a multiple-baseline single subject design, Kearns, Simmons, and Sisterhen (1982) were unable to attribute facilitation of verbal production to Amer-Ind training per se in two cases of aphasia without verbal apraxia. It appears, therefore, that the best candidates for Amer-Ind training for verbal facilitation have not yet been determined.

CONTEXT IN ACTION

This section focuses on some of the situations in which components of context cannot be easily separated. In these situations, a client has the opportunity to build confidence in his or her communicative ability when faced with variety and miscommunication. In addition, practice in the comprehension of speaker meaning may be approached with fairly structured tasks involving metaphor and other forms of context-dependent communication.

Conversation and Other Natural Interactions

We have been emphasizing the application of individualized contextual background to enhancing the meaningfulness of direct stimulation drill. Now, we wish to discuss more natural conditions for the practice of verbal and nonverbal communicative skills, especially conditions in addition to PACE discussed in the previous chapter. We want to stretch treatment beyond PACE so that an aphasic patient has an opportunity to practice behaviors that are unique to more natural conditions and an opportunity to practice trained skills in increasingly less secure circumstances. Furthermore, these situations still can be used to manipulate many specific contextual variables, such as topic (i.e., shared knowledge) and participant roles.

One guide to variety of circumstances is the numerous speech acts that are possible depending on the situation. A comprehensive list was provided by Wiig (1982) in a manual for developing social communicative competencies in pre-adolescents, adolescents, and young adults. A sampling of her list is provided in Table 5-2. Wiig's manual contains suggestions for setting up imaginary or role-playing situations in which these and other speech acts would be natural responses. With her target populations, Wiig could rely extensively on verbal instructions and the imaginations of her clients. She could somewhat directly instruct her clients to practice producing certain speech acts. With moderately to severely impaired aphasic individuals, on the other hand, we are limited to the need for arranging more concrete circumstances. For any activity, clinicians should *create communicative interactions in which varied speech acts are natural behaviors in such circumstances.*

Table 5-2. Wiig's (1982) List of Speech Acts*

Ritualizing (simple and elaborate, formal and informal)
  greetings
  farewells
  introducing oneself
  introducing another person
  request to repeat

Informing (simple and complex)   *Controlling* (direct and indirect)
  statement   wanting
  affirmation   offering
  denial   commanding
  rejection   suggesting
  evasion   promising
                                             warning
Feeling (direct and indirect)   assenting
  endearment   refusing
  exclamation
  approval
  disapproval
  congratulation
  apology

---

*This sampling is intended to be suggestive of the variety of purposes for which communicative behaviors might be used by a client in clinical interactions.

Eliciting Specific Speech Acts. As mentioned in Chapter 3, clinicians have arranged activities designed to assess production of particular speech acts. A prominent example is the stimulation of requests. At one point in the CADL (Holland, 1980), the client is required to write while the tester withholds a pencil. Hopefully the client will somehow ask for a pencil or pen. Prinz (1980) arranged several similar situations, such as offering a cigarette to subjects without providing a means to light it and offering a drink without indicating what is available. Clinicians might want to devise at least 10 such situations for practicing requests. However, there are a few problems with attempting to elicit at least other speech acts with such a treatment paradigm. First, improving the ability to produce speech acts is not necessarily a goal of treatment for aphasic persons. Research has shown that aphasic persons are able to convey a variety of intents, and the pertinent problem is that aphasic persons have difficulty with the linguistic mode of conveying a speech act. We want aphasic patients to use varied speech acts as a means of practicing linguistic skills for a variety of natural purposes. Therefore, focusing on one specific speech act may not be appropriate in aphasia treatment. Second, it is difficult to come up with at least 10 contrived situations that are not overly redundant or downright silly. What is best is to be cognizant of opportunities to elicit requests as well as other speech acts in situations that call for a variety of speech acts, such as role-playing a real-life activity. If an activity involves ordering in a restaurant, then withhold the menu. In this vein, the CADL does not consist of contrivances to elicit greetings and farewells. These intents are to be observed by the clinician in natural circumstances before testing begins and at the moment that it ends.

Simulated Life Situations. Clinicians often attempt to provide props or larger settings intended to simulate real-life communicative situations. The clinician may play roles of a store clerk or telephone operator, while the client imagines being in such situations. These activities should involve communication as a necessary component, as opposed to having the client do something and, then, encouraging him or her to talk about it. Schlanger and Schlanger (1970) described their activities with respect to pragmatic objectives: "What is needed. . . is the full use of this residual language and the development of compensatory communicative behavior to adjust to the changed language status" (p. 229). Just as Spradlin and Siegel (1982) recommended thinning the reinforcement schedule for treatment of children, simulated life situations provide a thinning of security normally found in direct stimulation. Simulations do not provide quick cues to bail the client out of trouble. Overcoming communication obstacles is practiced in these circumstances.

Schlanger and Schlanger (1970) divided their activities into nonstress situations (e.g., planning a picnic) and stress situations (e.g., going out to dinner). Stress situations included pleasant (e.g., going out to dinner) and unpleasant activities (e.g., emergencies or dealing with insensitive people). In all of these activities, a client played a role that would normally be assumed in these circumstances. An additional challenge was presented by having clients assume roles of people other than themselves in simulated situations. In general, situations should be based on a clinician's determination of current and potential contexts for communication. A patient may use any available means to communicate in these situations. For severely to moderately impaired patients, use of props is advisable in order to make the situation as concrete as possible. For patients with sufficient auditory comprehension, situations may simply be described verbally by the clinician who then asks the client to offer a likely response for the situation. Pictures are available that are intended to represent real life communication problems, as in Schlanger's *What's the Solution?* (1980) and her *Picture Communication Cards* (1978).

An aphasic patient may be led to participation in certain real life situations through the prior training of specific communicative skills that are inherent to a situation. In planning such training, a clinician should be realistic as to what is required communicatively (and not necessarily linguistically) in a situation. Ordering from a menu in a restaurant is a convenient example. While most aphasic persons would like to verbalize their orders, this goal may not be realistic at a particular point in a patient's recovery. Pointing to items, pictured or printed, achieves the same purpose. A patient can point to the word "steak" and practice saying "medium"; having to say both is unnecessary. Menus vary in their linguistic difficulty and in the extent that they provide pictured contexts. This variability in menus, obtained from restaurants in the area, can be built into a training program. Early training might entail a simple menu with many pictures, and a client may practice pointing to pictures and words to convey an idea. Reading items aloud can be encouraged. Then, it is important to practice these skills in a simulated situation, with a clinician playing the role of waiter or waitress. Even though a client may possess basic skills, in an actual situation the client still may not motion for the waiter or waitress to move into a position where he or she can see what the client is indicating.

Natural Conversation. Conversation has been considered a part of treatment strategy since the treatment of aphasia began. The thought of writing about how to engage in conversation seems to be silly; however, Wilcox and Davis (1977) and Kimbarow (1982) found a tendency for clinical conversations to resemble direct stimulation in terms of the speech acts produced (see Chapter 2). So, there appears to be a need to reconsider conversation as a therapeutic medium. We want to veer away from conversation such as the following:

> *Clinician:* "What did you do this weekend?"
> *Aphasic Person:* "Not much."
> *Clinician:* "Did you watch TV?"
> *Aphasic Person:* "Yes."
> *Clinician:* "Tell me what you watched."
> *Aphasic Person:* "The. . . series."
> *Clinician:* "You mean the World Series. Say, 'the World Series.' "
> *Aphasic Person:* "World Series."
> *Clinician:* "Good. Now, say, 'the World Series.' "
> *Aphasic Person:* "The. . . Series."
> *Clinician:* "Good. Who hit the home run?"
> *Aphasic Person:* "I know. I can't say it. Field, no. . . Field."
> *Clinician:* "You are close. Say, 'Winfield. . . Dave Winfield.' "

This conversation consists of a series of questions and requests by the clinician and answers from the aphasic participant. It contains two instances of what Kimbarow (1982) called "therapizing," that is, ignoring communicative success and pushing for linguistic virtuosity. Considering possible shared knowledge, the client's messages could have been conveyed. The clinician's behavior would not normally be tolerated in a conversation with a person without brain damage.

Wepman's (1972, 1976) content-centered discussion therapy offered perhaps the first guideline to yanking a clinician away from placing demands on linguistic precision during conversation with an aphasic adult. He suggested that conversation that focuses a client's attention on ideas of high individual interest is a legitimate treatment procedure that, in some cases, may result in improved verbal expression. Wepman considered that this improvement is the result of aiming treatment at a more appropriate primary deficit, namely, a limitation of thought processes. However, it is also possible that a reduction of attention to language processes and, therefore, of pressure on performance may be the mechanism that promotes improvement of linguistic performance.

Another guide to conceptualizing a conversation without unusual linguistic demands is simply to concentrate on maintaining natural conversation. The clinician may have to initiate an exchange with a question but then can offer statements, arguments, or other speech acts as a means of sustaining interaction on a topic. The clinician should be interested in the information that a client wishes to convey and should respond based on message conveyance whenever possible. The clinician should take a speaking turn for the purpose of conveying information or an opinion rather than for the purpose of eliciting better language.

When considering this perspective toward conversation with a patient, a conversation may proceed as follows:

> Clinician:"What did you watch on TV last night?"
> Aphasic Person: "The series."
> Clinician: "The World Series?"
> Aphasic Person: "Yes."
> Clinician: "I thought the Dodgers blew it."
> Aphasic Person: "No. Home run."
> Clinician: "Yes. I remember that. It was exciting. I don't remember who hit the home run."
> Aphasic Person: "Field, no. . . Field."
> Clinician: "Oh, yes. Dave Winfield. It was a long one, too."

As opposed to the previous example, the clinician makes more statements and renders more opinions. The clinician does attempt to elicit a name, but in a more natural manner. The patient's response is accepted as being communicative rather than as being inadequate. If improvement in retrieving names of baseball players is desired, then a formal task designed to exercise name retrieval (which, among many factors, controls for familiarity and ease of pronunciation) should be done. At some point, conversation should be preserved as conversation, in order to present a more natural condition in which language can be practiced. However, in considering the clinician's point of view, the ability to preserve naturalness of conversation depends on knowledge of a topic that is shared by the participants.

Speaker Meaning

In order to be comprehensive as to the communicative situations confronting an individual, a clinician may provide an opportunity for a client to practice nonliteral interpretation. The process of nonliteral interpretation appears to be relatively intact in moderately to mildly impaired patients, at least to the extent that it has been studied (see Chapter 2). However, traditional treatment has been focused solely on literal interpretation, with minimal attempt to create tasks in which meaning of an utterance is truly dependent upon a context in which it is used. Just as metaphor has been one communicative form that has been used to study the process of nonliteral interpretation, it may also be a vehicle for providing treatment exercises in this domain of pragmatic language behavior.

Our previous discussions of metaphor contain considerations that are useful in planning treatment exercises. The distinction between fresh and dead (i.e., idiom) metaphor is relevant, because dead metaphors appear to be processed similarly to literal interpretation. Fresh metaphors are unfamiliar relative to dead metaphors and often require attention to context in order to determine a speaker's intended meaning. Also, context-dependent metaphors, in which literal meaning of the utterance is plausible, demand attention to context for speaker meaning to be received. A problem for the clinician in planning a task is to present contexts along with the sentences to be used as metaphors. As mentioned earlier in this chapter, the pre-stimulation phase of a deblocking task may provide a proper paradigm for context presentation. A sentence may be preceded by a context that is either pictured or in verbal form depending on a patient's receptive abilities. Models for such tasks are found in the experimental literature cited in Chapters 1 and 2.

Another paradigm is found in the experimental literature with normal adults that indicates how stimulation of indirect request production might be achieved. It is similar to the story-completion task used by Helm-Estabrooks and coworkers (1981) for eliciting various syntactic forms. Gibbs (1981) designed a story-completion task in which the stories depicted situations that would naturally result in a request; his stories are listed in an appendix to his article. Normally, many of these requests would be produced indirectly if the listener were sensitive to social characteristics of the situations. The story-completion procedure is similar to the manner in which Wiig (1982) has developed tasks for the practice of a wider range of speech acts.

RETAINED LINGUISTIC CAPACITIES

Along with improving impaired verbal and other symbolic processes, the pragmatic clinician wishes to encourage greater use of retained linguistic behavior and competence. Some linguistic behaviors, while being classic symptoms of aphasic deficit, still communicate; and clincians have begun to turn away from discouraging any behavior that is a deviation and, instead, are now reinforcing the use of language that gets the idea across. We refer to competence, because sometimes a new modality is trained in order to give expression to dormant linguistic capacities.

Elaborating Retained Verbal Behavior

Adaptive or compensatory linguistic behaviors used by aphasic persons include word-finding strategies (Holland, 1982) and syntactic compensations of Broca's aphasia (Gleason et al., 1975). Communication obstacles of word-finding impairment are overcome with circumlocution, semantic paraphasias, spelling aloud, a request for time to verbalize, consulting a convenient word list, searching for objects, and so on. As discussed in Chapter 3, adaptation to agrammatism includes stressed opening words or "starters," adverbs to express time (instead of verb tense markers), and concatenation of phrases (instead of embedding). Persons with Broca's and moderate fluent aphasias may pause for a while before producing a word, or they may stop in the midst of an unsatisfactory production and start again. Many patients spontaneously repair their own utterances. They may request help from a listener. They may point out their message in a nearby book.

The first step in elaborating these strategies is to make the patient aware of their occurrence and of their communicative value. Increasing awareness can be achieved with traditional recognition paradigms. Patients with Broca's aphasia can practice recognizing grammatical errors in utterances presented by a clinician and in his or her own audio-recorded utterances. These patients are able to use their linguistic competence in order to recognize and correct errors (Bliss, Guilford, and Tikofsky, 1976). For other aphasic persons with serious comprehension deficits, awareness of communicative strategies may be achieved once direct treatment has improved comprehension ability. Realization of the communicative dividends of compensatory and self-correcting strategies often comes from experiencing their value in a new information condition, as in PACE therapy.

The next step has often been presented as an "encourage the use of" approach within the context of natural communicative interactions. Encouraging use entails simply reinforcing communicatively sufficient and adaptive behaviors whenever they occur. The criterion for desirable linguistic behavior should shift from the more traditional concern for linguistic precision to the more pragmatically oriented concern for communicative accomplishment. When a client says in conversation, "I took the train to the store," a clinician might respond with "I know what you mean, you took the bus" rather than with "No, that's wrong, you took the bus; say *bus*." A clinician should respond with comprehension to "I see doctor tomorrow" rather than interrupting discussion with an attempt to correct a patient's grammar. Furthermore, with respect to writing, the building-block approach to treatment might be avoided in that accurate spelling is not a prerequisite for a sentence to be understood. An accepting atmosphere should be created for whatever communicative linguistic behavior a patient is able to muster.

We are not recommending that objectives of word retrieval accuracy or sentence completeness be abandoned. Aphasic people who recognize their linguistic inaccuracies and imprecisions become frustrated and want to express themselves as they could before. We suggest that work on production of the best possible language be confined to traditionally structured tasks intended to facilitate the best possible response.

Giving Expression to Linguistic Capacities

In the search for alternative modes of communication for aphasic persons, teaching Amer-Ind may be one attempt to capitalize on retained symbolic capacities that can no longer be realized through speech. Speech is sometimes nearly impossible to elicit from aphasic persons who have severe apraxia of speech or who have global aphasia. Usually alternative means of communicating are developed for children and adults with motor speech disorders (e.g., Beukelman, Yorkston, and Dowden, 1985; Harris and Vanderheiden, 1980; McDonald, 1980; Owens and House, 1984). One alternative mode for expressing linguistic capacities includes *communication boards* and the small "tapewriters" with an alphabetized keyboard (Silverman, 1980). Clients require enough linguistic skill and motoric capacity to use such devices.

A fairly sophisticated communication board is the Handi-Voice 110, introduced in the treatment of a severely head injured adult by Warren and Datta (1981) nearly four years after onset. The Handi-Voice is a speech synthesizer that is activated by depressing a 128-cell, pressure sensitive grid.

A similar but smaller (and relatively inexpensive) device, called the Vocaid, has been produced by Texas Instruments. Warren and Datta described the achievements of their client: "After 7 months training, 3–4 hours per day, Jim was able to program complete sentences with the device. Spontaneously, he conversed in a telegraphic fashion, embellished by the use of memorized phrases or sentences" (p. 303). Moreover, after these several months of training with the Handi-Voice and about 56 months of virtually no functional speech, the client suddenly started talking. From a PICA verbal score of 4.75 at 35 months post onset, his score climbed to 13.15 at 60 months post onset. This aphasic individual, like many others trained in Amer-Ind, was described as having severe apraxia of speech. When this additional disorder makes it difficult for speech to be initiated, clinicians often turn to a new communicative mode. In some cases, it appears that the new mode may unlock a severely depressed speech mechanism.

Another category of new strategies consists of symbol systems not used before, such as Amer-Ind (Skelly, 1979) and Blissymbolics (e.g., Archer, 1977). *Artificial languages* were employed in investigations of cognitive abilities that might be retained in global aphasia. Based on a system developed for the chimpanzee, Glass, Gazzaniga, and Premack (1973) trained subjects with symbols varying in size, color, and shape that were functionally equivalent to words. Sentences could be formed by arranging the symbols from left to right on a table top. Learning at different stages of training was assessed by standard testing methods, such as selecting from two options the one that represented an object. Sentence level behavior involved following instructions, sentence completion, and arranging symbols in proper order. Two subjects were able to perform these tasks. The system was not evaluated as a means of communication in natural circumstances.

A similar system called Visual Communication (VIC) was developed "to circumvent the visual memory deficits and motor-coordination problems common in aphasia" (Gardner, Zurif, Berry, and Baker, 1976, p. 276). VIC's symbols were geometric shapes and representational drawings on small index cards. Some of the geometric shapes represented conjunctions and prepositions. Gardner's subjects were able to follow instructions presented in VIC, answer questions in VIC, and describe actions by the experimenter with these symbols. One subject used the system spontaneously to reveal his thoughts with statements and questions. After discharge from the hospital, his family continued the program at home. Both of these studies established the potential of such systems, but further investigation is needed regarding the functional application of such systems.

CHANGING COMMUNICATIVE CONTEXTS

Previously in this chapter, we have emphasized the manipulation of internal and external contexts as a means of changing the aphasic client's linguistic and other communicative behavior. In a sense, we have been concerned with bringing the client's world into the clinic in order to facilitate improvement of language function. Now our discussion turns to changing the client's world. This orientation is directed to the contexts themselves, without associating adjustments directly with the patient's communicative behavior. Lubinski (1981a, 1981b) referred to this arena of rehabilitation as "environmental intervention" with respect to a patient's internal and external environments. Other precedents include "environmental manipulation" for apraxia of speech (Florance, Rabidoux, and McCauslin, 1980) and "environmental education" for dysarthria in adults (Berry and Sanders, 1983).

Berry and Sanders (1983) stated that, in the management of dysarthria, direct treatment of impaired speech may or may not be appropriate, whereas environmental education can be implemented for nearly every dysarthric client. With respect to aphasic adults, we could advocate a similar position, especially when considering the discouraging results of language treatment for global aphasia. Furthermore, Kennedy (1983) considered environmental manipulation to be the only viable approach for Wernicke's aphasia. However, Wernicke's aphasia has been shown to possess mixed prospects for recovery (Kertesz and McCabe, 1977), and much more needs to be learned about the primary deficit of this disorder that may result in a sharper focus of direct treatment. Some changes can be accomplished in globally aphasic persons regarding their auditory language comprehension, and alternative modes of communication should be explored further. At least some attempt should be made to improve the communicative ability of every aphasic client. Yet, even with occasional failures in changing some patients, the modification of environmental factors in interpersonal communication can be rehabilitative for everyone.

Internal Contexts

Our first concern with respect to changing a patient's internal contexts pertains to treating impairments of semantic memory, usually in clients with severe auditory comprehension deficits. Our attack should be tentative, however, because of a lack of certainty as to whether such an impairment truly exists. Furthermore, when assuming that it does exist, there is a lack of certainty as to the nature of this impairment or, at least, as to the manner by which it should be characterized. Is it a disorganization of conceptual knowledge (therefore, demanding treatment of organization), or is it a "constriction" of semantic fields (therefore, demanding treatment that expands associations to a concept)? As with other treatments for rather newly discovered regions of deficit, we can appeal to basic research methodologies for suggesting exploratory treatments of semantic memory deficiency. These methods include sorting object-pictures into conceptual categories, associating pairs of objects related to each other on a number of different dimensions, and so on. More efficient access to conceptual knowledge may result in improved language comprehension, because essential language-context interactions may be improved.

Our second concern regarding internal context pertains to the psychological and emotional well-being of aphasic patients. A patient's internal psychological environment for treatment certainly influences readiness for hard work and possibly unusual modes of communication. While people react differently to life crises, certain regular stages of adjustment appear to occur subsequent to any type of loss (Tanner, 1980; Webster and Newhoff, 1981), and a patient's ability to adjust to "loss" of linguistic skill may depend on how easily he or she is progressing through these stages. Consultation with a clinical psychologist or psychiatrist may assist the clinician in covering this component of the pragmatic domain.

External Contexts

People in a client's everyday communicative environments are the most important contextual management targets not only because they can influence their communicative interactions with the client but also because they are often in a position to adjust the physical setting as well.

People. When dealing with family members, the clinician must touch indirectly upon marital relationships and family interaction patterns. These contexts are normally variable, and these persons have varied interest in and understanding of communication. Attempts to change communication strategies should begin at these multifarious starting points. Our recommendations are general and should be applied with flexibility according to adjustment needs, desires, and abilities. If changes in relationships themselves appear to be warranted, then referral to the appropriate professional is one means of changing context. For example, a positive attitude toward the client, in spite of communicative frustrations, certainly facilitates communicative interaction. This may be an easily achieved goal for a spouse in an already supportive marriage but may be an unrealistic expectation of a spouse for whom aphasia only exacerbates long-standing negative feelings. A marriage counselor may determine whether the marriage can be changed, while the speech-language pathologist considers this situation to be a given in anticipating whether changes in basic symbolic skills are likely to be accomplished.

Regarding communicative interaction, goals and procedures often are aimed at a hospital staff as well as family members, friends, or any other "significant other." The primary goal is *to maximize communication between conversational participants to the extent that communication occurred before onset of aphasia.* Meeting this goal does not necessarily entail the enforcement of changes in the nonaphasic communicative partner that did not already have to be made. A spouse, in particular, will have already had to figure out new ways of communicating and take on new responsibilities; and the clinical objective may be one of adjusting emotionally to such changes. Linebaugh, Kryzer, Oden, and Myers (1982) described a spontaneous shift to a greater-than-normal share of *communicative burden* assumed by a nonaphasic participant in conversations with an aphasic participant. Communicative burden is observed partly in the proportion of a conversation in which a participant must be the initiator of a specific interaction. Linebaugh defined one goal as adjusting to the burden of initiation by using this responsibility most effectively. Procedures would entail counseling and, perhaps, some training in effective communicative strategies.

Burden of the nonaphasic participant has been included in definitions of severity of impairment (Goodglass and Kaplan, 1972) and was found to be correlated with severity of communication deficit measured with the CADL (Linebaugh et al., 1982). As a listener, the nonaphasic partner does a great deal of guessing in the "hint-and-guess" sequence described by Lubinski and coworkers (1980). The nonaphasic partner assumes more responsibility than before onset in assisting the client in getting his or her idea across. Strategies for making most effective use of the receiver role are listed in Table 5–3. These suggestions involve attending to all contextual cues to a message, encouraging strategies trained in treatment, and being responsive with honesty. We believe that this third area stems simply from treating the aphasic person as an adult. It is likely that a family member is already following many or most of these suggestions. The clinician should observe interactions with the client and then work with the nonaphasic partner on areas that can be improved.

Table 5–4 provides suggestions for the nonaphasic partner in the role of sending messages to an aphasic person. As with enhancing the receiver role, the clinician should first observe the nonaphasic partner and then educate accordingly. Education or counseling can be enhanced if the partner is able to observe video recordings of interactions; he or she may often spontaneously recognize behaviors that should be modified. Towey

Table 5-3. Suggestions For Most Effective Use of Increased Communicative Burden in the Receiver Role

The Nonaphasic Receiver

Attend to all cues to the aphasic person's message. Be in a position to observe face and limb gestures.

Utilize physical setting and knowledge of prior events fully in order to realize the topic of the aphasic person's message. Persons outside the patient's family may have to assume an unusual responsibility in learning about what the patient knows.

Provide an accepting atmosphere for and reinforce use of strategies learned in treatment, even if they are imperfect linguistically.

Remind the aphasic person of strategies learned in treatment (e.g., timing gestures for verbal apraxia, pantomimes).

Give the aphasic person time to make a best effort to convey a message. Do not interrupt. Help when asked to do so or when frustration begins to mount.

Refrain from pretending to comprehend when you do not: Let the aphasic person know you do not understand and make a reasonable guess as to the message.

Refrain from pretending not to comprehend when you do: Reinforce the aphasic person's ability to get an idea across by indicating comprehension, instead of demanding more linguistic precision once a message has been conveyed.

Table 5-4. Suggestions For Most Effective Use of Increased Communicative Burden in the Sender Role

The Nonaphasic Sender

Use alerting signals, such as the aphasic person's name, when needed.

Minimize environmental noise that competes with attention to your message.

Talk to the aphasic adult like an adult. Be respectful.

Allow time for the aphasic person to comprehend.

Be ready to repeat, use pauses, or slow down when the aphasic person appears not to comprehend or when the aphasic person asks for such help.

Use simplified syntax or redundant wording, whichever helps.

Use words assumed to be known to the aphasic person.

Enhance your own supplemental cues, such as face and limb gesture. Try writing or drawing when appropriate.

and Pettit (1980) employed video recordings for training staff in a small rural rehabilitation hospital to interact most effectively with globally impaired individuals. Some partners may benefit from practice, occasionally in the structured interaction provided by PACE (e.g., Newhoff, Bugbee, and Ferreira, 1981).

Settings. Lubinski (1981a, 1981b) has discussed certain nursing home settings as being examples of "communication-impaired environments." Elements of a client's everyday physical settings may detract from achieving maximum communication with others. Lubinski reviewed four factors. *Lighting and visual cues* can be maximized for adequate perception of setting and communicative partners and for locating and identifying important areas in a building (e.g., use of color coding on doors and light switches). *Acoustic characteristics* of a room should facilitate speech perception, especially when an aphasic person has a hearing loss. An aphasic person should be able to control sources of noise. *Furniture arrangement* may discourage face-to-face communicative interaction. Circular arrangements indicate that interaction is permissible, and they facilitate use of nonverbal communicative modes. *Environmental props* may be used as supplemental cues to a topic of conversation or specific ideas. In an institutional setting, residents like to reach for personal items, mementos, and pictures to clarify a message. An aphasic person is most motivated to improve communicative skills when living in an environment in which interaction is frequent, available, and encouraged.

Finally, in addition to changing settings, treatment objectives can be framed around increasing the number of settings in which the client has opportunities to communicate and which provide topics of conversation later. Many clients have reduced the number of settings for communication since the onset of aphasia. They no longer visit friends, go to church, or attend sporting events. This change may be in response to linguistic and motoric limitations, and for some, it may occur because of a move to a more restricted environment such as a nursing home. Some of the suggestions earlier in this chapter, such as naturalizing task content and simulating life situations, may reduce a client's fear of recently shunned settings, as well as improve ability to communicate in them. People often do not respond to the mere suggestion to do this or that. An aphasic person in particular needs to feel confident that he or she can function in a situation before approaching it. By simulating situations, a clinician encourages a nursing home resident to participate in situations provided in the institution and in field trips of various kinds.

SUMMARY AND CONCLUSION

In this chapter we have attempted to extract treatment implications from the domain of pragmatics. While some of our suggestions might be novel to some clinicians, many clinicians will recognize that what they have been doing for their aphasic patients possesses relationships to different regions of pragmatics. A speech-language pathologist once remarked that she thought "legitimate" aphasia treatment is done at a table with line drawings of common objects and that, somehow, her work with home-bound clients in their kitchens is "illegitimate" treatment. Pragmatics seemed to provide the theoretical support that she needed to feel legitimate about working in a kitchen. However, the coverage of pragmatics consists of more than setting of treatment, and our model is designed to draw attention to all of the contextual variables that contribute to natural language behavior. These variables include linguistic, paralinguistic, and extralinguistic contexts, all of which influence the use of language in a conversational structure. In a variety of ways, these variables can be manipulated in direct and indirect approaches to treatment, so that an aphasic person can be exposed to the conditions under which he or she must function outside of the clinic.

Chapter 6

Treatment Implementation: Some Case Descriptions and Suggestions

In this chapter we want to further amplify our discussion of pragmatically oriented treatment. We have previously described the rationale as well as the general structure of the PACE interaction, including suggestions for adjusting PACE to meet the requirements of different levels and types of aphasia. We have also considered several issues relative to pragmatic treatment in general (see Chapter 5). At this time we want to focus on practical issues concerning the implementation of PACE and other pragmatic variables. We shall discuss aphasic clients with whom we have successfully used PACE as well as other pragmatically oriented treatment techniques. Although these cases cannot be regarded as formal research, the detailed clinical observations as well as pre- or posttesting provide convincing evidence relative to the importance or approaching treatment pragmatically. Finally, we shall consider group treatment for aphasic clients in terms of PACE and in a broader pragmatic perspective.

CASE DESCRIPTIONS

In the following sections it is our intention to provide a "nuts and bolts" description of pragmatically oriented treatment for aphasic adults. In Chapter 4 we discussed several issues pertaining to the adjustment of PACE for differing types and levels of aphasic impairment. The following case descriptions illustrate the technical implementation of the varying adjustment areas we suggested. Although in all cases we describe use of a PACE interaction, we also provide examples of treatment activities employing pragmatic issues discussed in Chapter 5. Initially, we shall present two cases focusing on individuals with a mild to moderate aphasia; we shall then discuss two cases demonstrating a more severe aphasia involvement; finally, we shall present a description of a PACE interaction occurring between two clients.

Mild to Moderate Aphasia

Case No. 1: Anomic Aphasia. Mary began treatment about two months after suffering a stroke at age 69. Her verbal behavioral patterns were such that a diagnosis of anomic aphasia was determined (Goodglass and Kaplan, 1972). As is typical of anomic aphasia, her verbal expression was fluent and grammatically complete, and she did not exhibit hemiparesis. Her moderate aphasia permitted her to retain fairly good conversation skills, inhibited primarily by word-finding difficulties. Her PICA overall score prior to treatment was at the 57th percentile (1981 norms), with auditory comprehension close to the normal range, reading at the 57th percentile, verbal expression at the 58th percentile, and writing at the same percentile. Her treatment was planned to improve word finding skills.

Prior to her stroke, Mary enjoyed playing bridge with a senior citizens' group that met once per week. She stopped playing bridge after her stroke, primarily because she used to drive herself and could no longer drive. Because of transportation difficulties, it was thought that Mary's return to the bridge group might be an unrealistic goal; but it was also thought that her interest in bridge might be employed in treatment where she could continue to enjoy this activity. Therefore, knowledge of bridge and playing bridge were considered to be vital horizontal contexts that would provide pragmatic content and procedures for treatment. One problem at the outset was that there was minimal shared knowledge of bridge between Mary and her clinician, because the clinician did not know how to play the game. Mary had to assume the role of teacher, and the clinician's preparation included reading a book about bridge.

Treatment was not intended to consist of simply playing bridge. Instead, the rules of the game served as topics of conversation, and analysis of the game led to creation of tasks that focused on specific features of the game. In this way, Mary practiced parts of bridge, one at a time, with each part requiring identifiable comprehension and expression abilities. For example, the clinician would display a hand, and Mary's task was to estimate the worth of her tricks in trump and no-trump situations. In order to challenge her expressive abilities, the clinician asked her to explain specific aspects of bridge, such as the point-count system used to determine the value of a hand.

Familiar card games can be the source of several standard stimulation activities. Many people enjoy playing poker. Word comprehension can be exercised by presenting a choice of hands and asking the client to point to the "straight" or the "flush." Conversely, word retrieval can be practiced by presenting a hand and asking the client to name it or describe it. Then, for natural interaction, the clinician and the client can play the game.

PACE was instituted in a way that encouraged Mary to rely on her linguistic strengths when faced with word retrieval problems. Pictures of objects were used in spite of her relatively high level of language ability. Instructions were given so that she could take advantage of her ability to circumlocute. She was asked not to concern herself with providing the name of the object and, in fact, was asked specifically not to give its name. Her task was to make the receiver (clinician) guess the object name from whatever other information that she could provide. Over a three week period, Mary's communicative efficiency rating in the PACE interaction improved from 3.7 to 4.0 to 4.2 with respect to the Davis (1980) 5-point rating scale.

During Mary's two months in treatment, her fluent expressive ability was measured once per week with a probe that required her to describe five pictures, each depicting multiple actions. Pictures of this complexity did not appear in treatment. With a multidimensional scoring system, expressive levels were measured at 90 per cent and 85 per cent over two weeks. These levels were too high to permit measurement of much improvement over time. Thus, a more difficult probe was needed. The new probe required Mary to produce procedural discourse, an activity that also was not contained in her treatment. She was asked to describe various procedures, such as how to make a sandwich. Her performance on each description was measured with a scale consisting of four points (a description with three elements in correct order) to zero points (no attempt). There was time to administer this probe only once, but her score did drop to a somewhat more desirable 75 per cent. At this point Mary became ill and treatment was discontinued. If Mary had not become ill, the clinician would have had to adjust the scoring system to produce a lower score and then readminister the probe several times to see if generalization of improvement could be demonstrated.

A second PICA was administered after these two months of treatment. Although Mary's improvement occurred within six months post onset (the spontaneous recovery period), the substantial changes in her test scores are of interest. The pre- and posttests were given by a clinician who did not provide the treatment. Overall, Mary's response level improved from 11.42 (57th percentile) to 13.37 (81st percentile). Her reading score improved from 11.90 to 14.50 and her verbal score from 12.03 to 13.60. The four writing subtest scores in the graphic section increased from 7.45 to 11.70.

Case No. 2: Anomic Aphasia. Again we address treatment of a mild to moderate disorder with characteristics of anomic aphasia (Goodglass and Kaplan, 1972). Finley was an enthusiastic conversationalist who had been employed as a machinist. At the age of 55, he was in an industrial accident in which his outerwear became entangled in a piece of machinery. His clothes were drawn into the machine, and he was strangulated for about 10 minutes. He suffered cerebral hypoxia, and five days later he had a marked language impairment resulting from obstruction of the left carotid artery.

About two months later a PICA revealed an overall score of 9.32 (34th percentile, 1981 norms). Just prior to beginning treatment, at three months post-onset, Finley's overall score was 11.00 (52nd percentile) with a verbal mean of 12.15 (59th percentile). During the next 10 weeks, he received direct stimulation and drills designed to improve auditory attention and comprehension, word-finding, reading, and spontaneous writing at the word level. Largely because of his continuing spontaneous recovery, his overall score improved further to 13.01 on the PICA (77th percentile). His verbal expression score was fluent and grammatically complete at 14.07 (85th percentile); and writing was occasionally in complete sentences. These scores represented a gain of 3.03 points over the previous test. Occasionally, when creative production of discourse was required, his syntax would become somewhat disorganized, indicative of a kind of paragrammatism found in fluent aphasias.

Finley was a good communicator verbally with little need for supplemental gesturing or writing in everyday conversation. The problems in planning PACE were to gear it toward his linguistic needs and to make it challenging enough so that it would be therapeutic. PACE was thereby employed so that Finley would exercise word retrieval for purposes of conveying new information; the clinician's turns as initiator or sender were seen as an opportunity for Finley to practice comprehension as well as word retrieval for confirming comprehension in his respondent or receiver role.

Selection of message stimuli was regarded as the crucial variable for adjusting the PACE procedure to this client's basic problem (word retrieval) and degree of impairment (mild). Pictures of common objects would have been too easy, so we decided to use pictures for less common words and printed words that encourage communication about abstract nonpicturable concepts. Sometimes the printed words were names of famous people.

The task was not simply to name the item. PACE was conducted somewhat like a Password game. Finley, in his turn as sender, was to give clues about the identity of the object or word on his message stimulus card. The clinician, as receiver, was to guess the identity of the object or word. The following is a script from a segment of one session; one notable feature of the interaction is Finley's participation in figuring out the clinician's message by asking questions (e.g., for Clark Gable). Also, famous people from Finley's earlier life were used.

Finley: (selects a card) "This man's name is the President of the. . . of this. . . of this, and I tried this before and it's a little trouble. This comes from Georgia."

Clinician: "Jimmy Carter."

Finley: "Jimmy."

Clinician: (selects a card) "This guy is a basketball player. He was player of the year."

Finley: "That is Bird."

Clinician: "Yep. Larry Bird."

Finley: "Larry Bird. Bird." (selects a card) "This is a lady who. . . who is in show biz here. . ."

Clinician: "Here in Memphis?"

Finley: "No. This is the larger scene. She is from. . . . She's a Limey lady, and. . ."

Clinician: "She's a what lady?"

Finley: "English woman. And his name, his husband is Burton."

Clinician: "Ah, Elizabeth Taylor. Her husband *was* Burton."

Finley: "Right."

Clinician: (selects a card) "This guy was a heartthrob back when you were a younger fella."

Finley: "Is he in show biz?"

Clinician: "In the movies."

Finley: "Is he a singer?"

Clinician: "No. He was in *Gone with the Wind*."

Finley: "That is a. . . Clark Grable. . . Gable."

Clinician: "Right."

Finley: (selects card) "This also was a lady who is very good, and I woulda liked to driven any of them, I suppose. And she. . . one job she does is Hush Hush in the Charlotte, Charlotte."

Clinician: "Oh, Bette Davis."

Finley: "Good. And I'm a gonna miss them people."

One of the ingredients in PACE that makes it so similar to natural conversation is the active part played by the receiver in determining whether the sender's message is conveyed. An aphasic sender does not attempt to communicate in a vacuum outside of the clinic. A receiver must pay attention and sometimes formulate guesses based on partial information. Occasionally, in natural conversation, a listener's success in comprehending is just a lucky guess. The only time message conveyance is up to the speaker alone is during traditional confrontation naming or picture description drills. Therefore, in PACE the clinician should pay attention and formulate guesses based on the information given by the client. Sometimes the clinician may take a little longer than someone else might have taken to figure out a client's message. This ability to understand may vary as a function of the clinician's alertness, knowledge of the topic, and other factors found in natural communicative contexts. This point is illustrated in the next segment of a session with Finley:

> Finley: (selects a card) "This is a written record of a. . . an account in a store, because you can be sure that they will fund it you don't."
> Clinician: "A refund?"
> Finley: "He will not refund unless you have this little piece of paper and it goes in your package."
> Clinician: "On the package?"
> Finley: "It goes in the bag. The first thing you throw in here is this piece of paper that has a written record."
> Clinician: "For the sale?"
> Finley: "That's right."
> Clinician: "The receipt."
> Finley: "Yes."
> Clinician: (selects a card) "It comes in a spray or roll-on."
> Finley: "Deodorant."
> Clinician: "Yes."
> Finley: (selects a card) "Some people use the pick and. . . pick and peck type. Some people use only the peck and punch method."
> Clinician: "To type, typing?"
> Finley: "Yeah. How's that for you?"
> Clinician: (selects a card) "You use them in here, to clean your teeth." (gesturing as if picking teeth)
> Finley: "This is fross, fross, dental fross, sauce. . ."
> Clinician: "Well. . ."
> Finley: "Fross. I can't say that word."
> Clinician: "That's. . . I'd better give you another clue. Um. . ."
> Finley: "Is it wood?"
> Clinician: "Yeah. It's wood."
> Finley: "It's a. . . It's a pick. . . pick, uh toothpick."
> Clinician: "Yeah, toothpick. That's right."
> Finley: "Toothpick."

Upon reviewing the preceding script, one might think that with "receipt" the clinician could have guessed correctly, based upon the information provided by Finley, at a sooner point than she did. This "delayed correct guess" is probably attributable to receiver alertness or familiarity and provides a good example of issues raised in Chapters 4 and 5 relative to receiver variability. That is, some receivers seem to function more efficiently and effectively than others. Also, the same receiver frequently demonstrates varying skills. We are not particularly concerned about receiver variability, as it is reflective of natural communicative contexts in which everyone is subject to variability with respect to listening skills.

The "toothpick" example of the script demonstrates another dynamic of the PACE interaction. In this portion, Finley's desire to comprehend accurately (along with the clinician's slightly ambiguous clue) compelled him to provide his own clue once he realized that his first guess was incorrect. This example illustrates the mini-turn sequence described in Chapter 4. In such sequences, minor communicative role reversals (i.e., client originally functions as receiver but assumes sender role while communicating about a particular topic) occur because the process of conveying a given message is a joint effort.

Another component of Finley's treatment illustrates the pragmatic approach to activities presented in Chapter 5. We wanted him to practice comprehension and expression that would be required in his natural communicative settings. One setting involved a return to work, a possibility that was strongly supported by his employer. However, Finley would return as a worker in a warehouse where he would be receiving and giving instructions as to the placement of objects on shelves. An artificial activity was constructed in the clinic so that he could practice this type of language use. Materials included small blocks of different shape, color, and size. Finley followed the clinician's instructions for arranging the blocks, and then the clinician followed his instructions. The task proceeded from simple to complex arrangements and began with duplicate sets of blocks in full view of both participants. Therefore, Finley could arrange his own blocks as he instructed the clinician in the manner in which to arrange her blocks. Subsequently, a partition between the clinician and client was introduced, thereby prohibiting the clinician's view of Finley's arrangement of blocks. This injected the dynamic of new information into the drill, demanding that Finley be more precise in his verbal instructions.

Finley returned to work in the warehouse. His PICA scores continued to improve, but less dramatically during this 8 to 11 month period after onset. After a slight drop in scores following a six week absence from treatment, his overall score improved to 13.42 (82 percentile). His gestural score (including auditory and reading comprehension) improved from 12.33 to 13.74 during this period, and his verbal expression leveled off with scores of 13.45 and 13.69.

Severe Aphasia

Case No. 3: Wernicke's Aphasia. Tom was a severely impaired individual with Wernicke's aphasia. His first PICA overall score, six months after onset, was 8.14 at the 23rd percentile (1981 norms). Until this time, treatment had been focused on improving attention to auditory stimuli and developing an ability to make appropriate responses to discrete auditory input. Meeting these objectives required a decrease in press for speech during auditory stimulation. For the next 18 months, treatment involved stimulation of comprehension and self-monitoring of verbal production improved, and neologistic jargon ceased. His overall score improved to 9.83, and his gestural summary score improved from 10.05 to 13.65 during this 18 month period. His verbal score continued to hover around 5.00. Then, Tom started to repeat components of auditory input, and from that point the clinician was able to elicit meaningful verbalization. During the next year, he achieved a verbal score of 8.33 and an overall score of 10.86.

PACE had not been developed until midway into Tom's treatment program. Even at this time, his processing difficulties were so great that we preferred maintaining a program consisting primarily of highly structured drills that would maximize comprehension. Also, we were finding that a time-consuming deblocking program was facilitating verbalization. Treatment did include training in the use of gesture and a notebook of printed words as alternative modes of communication. Finally, PACE was instituted in order to encourage use of gesture, use of the notebook, and some verbal production to convey messages in a more natural conversational structure. PACE was particularly useful for this client, because its structure of turn-taking forced Tom to practice listening during his turn as receiver, and allowed him to use his communication channels as a receiver and sender of messages. It also provided a structure in which Tom and his wife could practice communicating, with his use of the supplemental channels.

We wish to use the following dialogues from PACE to illustrate interaction between Tom and his wife (Virginia). Message stimuli consisted of pictures of common objects. In her turn as sender, Virginia was to use gestures and verbal clues to the object name so that Tom's turn as receiver could be an opportunity to practice word retrieval:

> Tom: (selects a card) "Wing. Wing." (shows her his card)
> Virginia: "Ring."
> Tom: "Ring."
> Virginia: "Yes." (selects a card) "You tell time by this, but it's a. . ."
>   (gestures a large shape)
> Tom: "Watch, watch."

Virginia: "No, (gesturing a large shape), it sits on a mantle or a shelf. Its larger than a watch."
Tom: "Uh, uh. . ."
Virginia: "Clock."
Tom: "Pick. Tock. Pock. Wock."
Virginia: "Clock. Uh, hum. . . that's pretty good."
Tom: (selects a card, gestures a motion around his face and neck)
Virginia: "Oh, I know. Perfume."
Tom: "Hoo. . . spoo. . . ter. . . spoo."
Virginia: "Perfume. . ." (nodding in agreement)
Tom: "Per. . . pume."
Virginia: "Perfume. That's good." (selects a card, and then gestures with left hand beside her ear and with right hand making a dialing motion)
Tom: "Hello? Virginia?"
Virginia: (nods affirmatively) "What do I have in my hand? What am I talking through?"
Tom: "Hello."
Virginia: "What is it?"
Tom: "Hello. . . uh. . . phone, phone, phone."
Virginia: "Yes."
Tom: (selects a card) "Uh. . . (reaches toward his feet) uh. . . socks, socks."
Virginia: "Socks. Yes, OK." (selects a card and points to her glasses)
Tom: (reflectively reaches for his glasses) "That's a. . . uh. . . what is it?"
Virginia: "Glasses."
Tom: "Grasses, glasses. Glasses." (selects a card) "Bah, bow, boat. . . hoat, coat! Hoat, coat." (shows her the picture)
Virginia: "Yes, its a long coat."
Tom: "Long. . ."
Virginia: "Long coat."
Tom: "Long. . ."

Upon examining the preceding script it can be seen that the mini-turns in this interaction tended to occur rapidly because of Tom's frequently quick responses to Virginia. Some of Tom's responses were reflexive, such as "Hello" in response to Virginia's phoning gesture. On his first turn as sender, Tom broke one rule of the PACE game by showing his card before completion of the communication. He refrained from doing this again. On Virginia's turn with "clock," she gave him the answer before he had much of a chance to convey his comprehension. Occasionally, both participants worked briefly on linguistic adequacy of Tom's verbalizations as in ("perfume" or "long coat"). Overall, this series of interactions demonstrates a series of successful communications.

We shall provide a scripted segment from one more interaction with Virginia, when the message stimuli were changed from pictures of objects to pictures of simple actions. With these pictures, Tom is free to use any channel to convey any element of the picture. Even though in PACE the client is not instructed to verbalize, this client produced several different words in the interaction:

> Tom: (selects a card) "Car. . . uh. . . car. . ."
> Virginia: "Give me. . ."
> Tom: "Car. It's a car. Water. Water. Girl. Two of them."
> Virginia: "What are they going to do to the car?"
> Tom: "Water. . ."
> Virginia: "Wash. Washing the car."
> Tom: "Yes."

In the above sample, although it is obvious that Virginia would have liked to have heard the verb or even a complete sentence, she made a reasonable inference, based on the information given, and communication was achieved. Finally, during another one of Tom's turns as sender, he spontaneously pulled his notebook from his pocket when other communicative channels failed him. After three guesses by Virginia that Tom rejected, she asked for another clue. Tom searched his notebook until he found the word "pot" to convey what was on a stove.

It is very likely that Tom and Virginia would have developed some sort of satisfactory communication system on their own, without the benefit of PACE. However, it was our overall impression that PACE provided an opportunity for Virginia to experience many communicative successes with Tom via channel combinations. It is our observation that sometimes spouses may tend to rely too heavily on single channels, particularly the verbal channel and may also tend to overemphasize verbal perfection. Experience in a PACE interaction may facilitate recognition of the importance of conveying a message (rather than linguistic accuracy), as well as allowing first-hand experience with communicative successes associated with nonverbal channels and channel combinations.

Case No. 4: Global Aphasia. The most severely impaired aphasic clients have often been disconcerting for the speech-language pathologist, primarily because recovery of speech and language functions has been poor, and traditional direct stimulation techniques have had little impact on recovery of impaired functions. Furthermore, many clinicians might be discouraged about using PACE, because severely impaired clients may appear to possess few communicative strengths that can be employed in the procedure. Nevertheless, globally impaired aphasic persons retain some nonverbal vehicles for communication, and they can improve their auditory comprehension and gestural skills (Sarno and Levita, 1981).

PACE creates an opportunity for a severely impaired client to (a) practice alternative modes of communication that have been identified by the clinician as being in use by the client, (b) discover modes of communication that are not currently being used, and (c) practice using skills in comprehension and expression in a somewhat natural situation. With the client to be discussed here, PACE was manipulated in a way that produced verbalizations that had not been achieved with other forms of treatment.

Cleatus suffered a left hemisphere thrombosis at age 57, five months prior to beginning a comprehensive language treatment program. He had a PICA overall score of 8.34, at the 25th percentile (1981 norms). His auditory comprehension was at 11.80 (25th percentile), and his verbal expression was at 7.32 (32 percentile). Verbal behavior was demonstrated as repetitions of single words. Cleatus was unable to read, as evidenced by a score of 5.00 (7th percentile). He had right hemiplegia and slight malformation of the left hand due to a viral infection. Overall, Cleatus had essentially no functional speech and had reduced dexterity with his only usable hand when treatment began.

PACE was introduced early in treatment in order to demonstrate to Cleatus that he was capable of communicating. Because he was without speech, writing, and a facile gestural mode, the clinician's task was to figure out modes by which Cleatus could convey a message to someone. He was able to recognize pictures of objects, and he could point with his left hand. Therefore, pointing to pictures, as if he were using a picture book as a communication aid, was the viable choice for an expressive channel. Because of Cleatus' low level of auditory comprehension, the clinician had to keep her messages simple. Cleatus was required to point to a set of pictures to indicate his comprehension. With these considerations, we had an initial plan for the PACE interaction:

>Message Stimuli: Object pictures
>Clinician's Model: Object name and pointing to picture
>Client's Channels: Pointing to pictures

Cleatus and the clinician were seated facing each other with a stack of object pictures on the table between them. A duplicate set of eight pictures (called the "response set") was face-up to Cleatus's left so that he could point to them easily. The clinician took the first turn as sender by selecting a message stimulus and then stating the object name and pointing to its picture in the response set. Cleatus indicated comprehension by simply pointing to the same picture in the response set. Cleatus took a turn as sender by selecting a message stimulus and pointing to the corresponding picture in the response set. Thus, all Cleatus needed to do was to match pictures. However, this ability was put to use in a communicative framework provided by the principles of PACE. At a very simple level, matching pictures resulted in success for Cleatus in communicating. The difficulty of PACE was increased slightly by making the pictures in the response set similar to, instead of duplications of, the message stimuli. Also, demands on Cleatus's word comprehension ability were increased by the clinician's stating the object name without pointing in her turn as sender.

After the preceding adjustments were made we noticed that when Cleatus pointed to a picture to indicate comprehension he frequently said the object name. Within a week (four sessions) he became verbal as a receiver but was still nonverbal as a sender. We decided to veer away from the PACE principles slightly by "stacking the deck" in order to encourage transfer of verbal behavior as a receiver to verbal behavior as a sender.

The deck of message stimuli was stacked so that a picture selected by the clinician in her turn as sender would be repeated when, subsequently, Cleatus took his turn as sender. With this arrangement, he would have just stated the word as a receiver that he would want to express as sender. After only a couple of sessions Cleatus was recognizing that he had just said the needed word as receiver. Following this recognition he began to say the word in his turn as sender in order to convey a message. In effect, we tricked him into utilizing his repetition ability within the context of conversational interaction. Within a couple of additional sessions, we no longer resorted to stacking the deck, and Cleatus began attempting to verbalize, instead of pointing to pictures, when serving as sender. Also he began attempting more gesturing with his left hand. Direct imitation training was instituted in an attempt to reduce the vagueness of his gestures.

Cleatus's progress, as described above, occurred during his first three weeks of treatment (12 sessions). Once Cleatus began verbalizing and gesturing, we removed the "response set" of pictures, and PACE proceeded with reliance on verbal and gestural channels. While Cleatus never surpassed the single word level of verbal production, by seven months post onset he had some functional verbal behavior, whereas two months previously he had had none.

Cleatus's verbal PICA scores improved between the fifth and seventh months post onset from 7.32 to 9.05. He achieved his highest verbal score of 12.13 nine months later as he named eight of the 10 objects. His overall score improved from 8.34 (25th percentile) to 10.56 (42nd percentile) during this 11 month period. His primary mode of communicating became single words, accompanied only occasionally by a helpful gesture. Attributing this improvement solely to PACE would be difficult, because Cleatus received direct stimulation of auditory comprehension, verbal expression, and gesturing in addition of PACE. However, it was within the PACE interaction that he began to verbalize spontaneously in order to convey a message.

PACE: Between Two Clients

One extralinguistic variable having an influence on communicative behavior is the participants in a conversational interaction. In Chapter 2 we discussed some pilot investigations, in which an aphasic client has been a constant, while partners have been varied to include spouses and familiar and unfamiliar clinicians. PACE provides a structured interaction in which (a) the influence of this variable on the ability to convey new information can be studied or (b) this variable can be used to vary the circumstances in which a client can practice communication skills for therapeutic purposes. We shall describe a PACE interaction between a client with anomic aphasia and one with apraxia of speech. The unusual feature about this pairing of partners is that either one could be considered the constant or the variable. One is providing a different and challenging context for the other.

Mary, discussed in an earlier case presentation, was the partner with anomic aphasia. She had good auditory comprehension at a PICA level of 14.60. Her verbal expression was fluent, at a level of 12.03. James, on the other hand, was nonfluent with a mild to moderate aphasia and a marked apraxia of speech that had been improving steadily for over a year. At the time of his PACE interaction with Mary, his PICA overall score was 12.32 (68th percentile), his auditory comprehension was at 15.00, and his verbal score was at 12.68. He was able to retrieve all object-names on the PICA with performance being held back primarily by his apraxia of speech and some agrammatism.

Each client introduced communicative challenges for the other in the context of the PACE interaction. For both, the new information component was strengthened because neither client was particularly familiar with the message stimuli used by the other. Mary, when serving as sender, had to adjust her verbal expression so that she could convey her messages to James, whose comprehension ability was somewhat less than that of a clinician (6 out of 12 for complex material on the Boston Diagnostic Aphasia Examination). James placed additional communicative burden on Mary, because he was less inclined than a clinician to make guesses about her messages because of his verbal limitations. As a receiver, Mary had to sharpen her listening in order to respond appropriately to James. Also, she exercised her word finding skills in the conversational function of guessing another's message when it was incomplete. James, when serving as sender, was forced to sharpen his articulatory accuracy for a mildy aphasic listener. As a receiver, he had an opportunity to try out his improving articulation in order to produce guesses when Mary's messages were unclear. Let us examine some segments of Mary and James' PACE interaction, as illustrations of these points:

> James: (selects card) "Uh, uh, here." (cutting motion with fingers)
> Mary: "Scissors?"
> James: "Yeah."
> Mary: (selects card) "Now, uh (pounding table with her fist) and um. . . I don't know. This takes some nails."
> James: "Oh. A ham. . . hammer."
> Mary: "Yeah."

In the preceding example, both participants used gestures to convey messages, with Mary combining gestural and verbal channels. Both were successful at retrieving and articulating words as receivers in order to make a guess about a message. Both had an opportunity to practice responding to guesses. In the following segment, James's auditory precision was tested:

> James: (selects card) "Uh, uh, here." (pretends to write)
> Mary: "Uh. . . pen?"
> James: "No."
> Mary: "Pencil?"
> James: "Yeah."

In this brief example of mini-turns, James had to analyze and respond to Mary's guess. Mary had to retrieve two slightly different words in an effort to convey her comprehension to James.

In the next segment, Mary takes some time to get to a meaningful "hint" about the message stimulus:

> Mary: (selects card) "An um. . . you don't see these. Yeah they do. Let me see. What else can I tell about? What kind of transportation in the air?"
> James: "Oh. . . an airblane, plane."
> Mary: "Okay."

In spite of Mary's awkward phrasing, James was concerned only about the message. He spontaneously improved his articulation as he also reinforced Mary's success as a communicator.

Both participants may produce varied words during the several mini-turns it can sometimes take for a message to be conveyed. Following is an example of such variance:

> James: (selects card) "News and movies. . . uh, news, movies" (turning motion with hand, and sits back with hands on chest pretending to watch something)
> Mary: "Movies?"
> James: "Yeah, movies, news, five. . ."
> Mary: "Um. . . that's hard."
> James: "Alright." (turning motion with hand)

Mary: "Turn it on."
James: "Yeah." (pretending to watch something again)
Mary: "Watch."
James: "Uh-huh."
Mary: "Television."
James: "Yeah!"

As a final note concerning an interaction between two clients, these two participants communicated a special interest in each other, perhaps because each could empathize with the problems of the other. They encouraged each other, and even provided some gentle ribbing that might be comfortable only in the following circumstance:

Mary: (selects card) "And this is uh. . . you wear it and. . . my son never
          takes it off regardless of. . ."
James: "Ring?"
Mary: (shakes head negatively)
James: (a gestural request for more information)
Mary: "Let's see. . . they don't have one in this room, but. . ."
James: "Watch?"
Mary: "Watch, yes. I thought you were *never* gonna get it."

GROUP TREATMENT

The term "group treatment", by itself, means no more than simply the treatment of more than one client in one session. Just as individual treatment varies as a function of goals and procedures, group treatment also may vary according to differing goals and respective procedures. This point is an important one, because to a few speech-language pathologists "group treatment" involves only certain goals and formats. For example, some may think of it only as a coffee break or informal social time, and others may think of it only as psychotherapy. However, there are as many objectives for group treatment as there are objectives for treatment in general.

One objective of group treatment is the same as the objective of pragmatic treatment in general and of PACE in particular. That is, group treatment can be employed as a special means of improving an aphasic person's ability to participate in a conversation. Furthermore, our discussion of group methodology shall focus on planned activity that includes a pragmatic orientation whereby the principles of PACE are easily incorporated. Our guidelines for creating activities for groups are as follows:

1.   The activity should be one in which communication is necessary for the activity's goals to be accomplished. This contrasts with having

the clients do something and then just encouraging them to talk about what they are doing or why they are doing it.

2. The clients should be able to interact with each other. The activity should be constructed so that the clinician is not an essential participant. The clinician's role should be to facilitate interaction or assist a client only when the interaction is disrupted or halted. This facilitates client communicative functioning in an independent and spontaneous manner.

3. Materials should be arranged so that the participants are conveying new information to each other.

4. Participants should take turns initiating an interaction, with each having an equal number of initiation opportunities.

5. Each participant should have the opportunity to communicate successfully. Therefore, the activity should be structured so that each client can choose whatever communicative channel that is functional. If one of the participants uses a notebook, for example, the activity should be such that the notebook can be used.

6. The activity should be kept simple, so that participants are not distracted by the activity itself. Minimal time should be spent on instructions for the activity or on learning the activity.

We generally try to construct activities that represent real-life situations or that simply are pure fun. Adults enjoy activities in which the goal is to score the most points or complete a task first. Cooperation may be incorporated into a competitive activity when, in a group of four clients for example, the participants can be paired into teams. Finally, whenever we have an idea for an activity, these guidelines become a checklist, and the activity is molded so that it conforms to each point on the list. Probably the most common type of activity that we use is some form of game, and in the following sections we describe two games and other less game-like activities. Our discussions of group activity types do not represent new information for many clinical aphasiologists. Our intent is not so much to provide new information as it is to clinically discuss ways in which group treatment can incorporate pragmatic aspects of communication.

Two-of-a-Kind

This is a simple card game in which the cards consist of duplicate sets of object pictures. Each client is dealt a hand of five cards, and the remaining cards are placed in a single stack in the middle of the table. The clients take turns attempting to obtain a match for one of the cards they are holding. This is done first by requesting a card from another player; then if that player does not have the card, the initiator must draw a card from the stack. Each time a match is obtained, the picture pair is removed from the hand. The goal is to obtain enough matches to be the first player without any cards left in the hand.

In the above activity each group guideline is followed. First, communication is necessary, because each player must request a particular card from another player. Saying the other player's name is also encouraged. The other player must also make a response. Second, the structure of the game requires that players interact with each other, while the clinician is not one of the players. Third, hands held in the card game are message stimuli hidden from view of the other players so that the new information principle is preserved. Fourth, turn-taking is part of the game. Fifth, players may request an object through any communicative channel of their choosing. Sixth, this is a simple card game that is familiar to many people, and in subsequent sessions, the rules usually do not have to be reviewed. Players can concentrate on communicating their requests for matching cards. The game can be varied by changing the content of the cards.

Picture Bingo

Each player is given a bingo card with pictures on it instead of numbers. A stack of individual stimulus cards is used for calling out the item to be covered on the bingo card. These stimulus cards may be pictures, or they may be printed words expressing the object name or function depending on the level of the group. Each player takes a turn selecting a stimulus card and then conveying the item to the others. If the item appears on their cards then it is covered with a small token (e.g., poker chip). The game ends when the first player covers all spaces on his or her card.

With the bingo activity, all group guidelines are followed. First, communication is necessary. Second, the clients play the game with each other. Third, each stimulus item is viewed only by the player calling out the item. Fourth, the players take turns. Fifth, the stimulus item may be conveyed in any channel. Sixth, it is a simple and familiar activity. As with any group activity, picture bingo should be adjustable to each participant's linguistic abilities. In this game, some players may call out items from object pictures, and other players may call out items from printed descriptions of object function.

Other Group Activities

Group activities not taking a game format may include cooperative efforts in planning a particular project or role-playing situations in which each participant carries out a predetermined function. One activity we have used is the planning of a vacation. Each participant takes a turn suggesting ideas related to certain components of a vacation plan, such as where they want to go, how much they are willing to spend, how they want to get there, what they want to take with them, and so on. Asking the group to agree on each topic promotes a variety of speech acts such as arguing and warning.

An idea for a role-playing activity arose one day when there was a large fire a few blocks from the clinic, its plumes of smoke being visible for several miles. Each client was capable of some verbalization, and so the activity involved use of the telephone. Each client was asigned a role relative to the event of the fire. One client was the first to observe the flames and had to make an emergency call to an operator. Another client was the operator, who then had to call the fire department's dispatcher. Another client was the dispatcher, who then had to notify the fire fighters.

Group treatment may be carried out with goals that are similar to those for individual treatment. Yet, as can be seen with the preceding examples of activities, group treatment possesses characteristics that are not attained in individual treatment, therefore making it a valuable supplement to individual treatment (Davis, 1983). The mutual support and encouragement that clients provide each other is derived largely from the empathy that aphasic individuals have for each other. It is a quality of empathy that the nonaphasic clinician cannot possess. Also, the language impairments of each participant provide unique challenges for each client in comprehending and conveying messages. Because they function somewhat independently and are able to assist each other, they may find increased confidence in their communicative abilities. Furthermore, group treatment provides the clinician with an opportunity to observe the potential fruits of individual treatment in a different communicative setting. It is another chance to promote and, hopefully, to observe generalization of individual treatment gains.

CONCLUSION

In presenting our suggestions in Chapters 5 and 6, we accomplished the sixth and final step of our progression of treatment development that was introduced in Chapter 1. With respect to our fourth and fifth steps, some procedural considerations have already been studied extensively in that our implications from pragmatics pertain to the semantic content and addition of variables in standard stimulation and behavior modification methodology. With the words of Rosenbek (1979), our feet might become more wrinkled with comparisons between standard content and more individualized content in such procedures. The suggestions that appear novel, such as PACE or conversational strategies, should be investigated further as to their effectiveness in helping patients communicate better. Most treatment procedures need to be scrutinized with respect to their impact on natural communicative behavior, the measurement of which has been elusive. The assessment suggestions of Chapter 3 should stimulate further development of measures that determine the outcome of treatment. We are confident that there are more implications of the pragmatic domain for treatment than are mentioned here, especially implications that become evident as more is learned about the relationships between language behavior and contexts. We are similarly confident that speech-language pathologists will use their understanding of pragmatics to provide us with what might be missing.

References

Apel, K., Newhoff, M., and Browning-Hall, J. (1982, November). *Contingent queries in Broca's aphasia*. Paper presented at the annual meeting of the American Speech-Language-Hearing Association, Toronto.

Archer, L. (1977). Blissymbolics — A nonverbal communication system. *Journal of Speech and Hearing Disorders, 42*, 568-579.

Bandura, A., and Harris, M. (1966). Modification of syntactic style. *Journal of Experimental Child Psychology, 4*, 341-352.

Barnes, G. (1983). Suprasegmental and prosodic considerations in motor speech disorders. In W. Berry (Ed.), *Clinical dysarthria* (pp. 57-68). San Diego: College-Hill Press.

Basso, A., Faglioni, P., and Spinnler, H. (1976). Non-verbal colour impairment of aphasics. *Neuropsychologia, 14*, 183-193.

Baum, S., Daniloff, J., Daniloff, R., and Lewis, J. (1982). Sentence comprehension by Broca's aphasics: Effects of some suprasegmental variables. *Brain and Language, 17*, 261-271.

Bear, D. (1983). Hemispheric specialization and the neurology of emotion. *Archives of Neurology, 40*, 195-202.

Berndt, R., and Caramazza, A. (1980). A redefinition of the syndrome of Broca's aphasia: Implications for a neuropsychological model of language. *Applied Psycholinguistics, 12*, 225-278.

Berry, W., and Sanders, S. (1983). Environmental education: The universal management approach for adults with dysarthria. In W. Berry (Ed.), *Clinical dysarthria* (pp. 203-216). San Diego: College-Hill Press.

Beukelman, D., Yorkston, K., and Dowden, P. (1985). *Communication augmentation: A casebook of clinical management*. San Diego: College-Hill Press.

Beukelman, D., Yorkston, K., and Waugh, P. (1980). Communication in severe aphasia: Effectiveness of three instructional modalities. *Archives of Physical Medicine and Rehabilitation, 61*, 248-251.

Black, J., and Bern, H. (1981). Causal coherence and memory for events in narratives. *Journal of Verbal Learning and Verbal Behavior, 20*, 267-275.

Bliss, L., Guilford, A., and Tikofsky, R. (1976). Performance of adult aphasics on a sentence evaluation and revision task. *Journal of Speech and Hearing Research, 19*, 551-560.

Blumstein, S., and Goodglass, H. (1972). The perception of stress as a semantic cue in aphasia. *Journal of Speech and Hearing Research, 15*, 800-806.

Blumstein, S., Goodglass, H., Statlender, S., and Biber, C. (1983). Comprehension strategies determining reference in aphasia: A study of reflexivization. *Brain and Language, 18*, 115-127.

Boller, F., Cole, M., Vrtunski, P., Patterson, M., and Kim, Y. (1979). Paralinguistic aspects of auditory comprehension in aphasia. *Brain and Language, 7*, 164-174.

Bond, S., Ulatowska, H., Macaluso-Haynes, S., and May, E. (1983). Discourse production in aphasia: Relationship to severity of impairment. In R. Brookshire (Ed.), *Clinical Aphasiology Conference proceedings* (pp. 202-210). Minneapolis: BRK Publishers.

Britton, B., and Tesser, A. (1982). Effects of prior knowledge on use of cognitive capacity in three complex cognitive tasks. *Journal of Verbal Learning and Verbal Behavior, 21*, 421-426.

Brookshire, R. (1978). *An introduction to aphasia* (2nd ed.). Minneapolis: BRK Publishers.

Brookshire, R., and Nicholas, L. (1984). Comprehension of directly and indirectly stated main ideas and details in discourse by brain-damaged and non-brain-damaged listeners. *Brain and Language, 21*, 21-36.

Brown, B., Strong, W., and Rencher, A. (1974). Fifty-four voices from two: The effects of simultaneous manipulations of rate, mean fundamental frequency, and variance of fundamental frequency on ratings of personality from speech. *Journal of the Acoustical Society of America, 55*, 313-318.

Brown, P., and Fraser, C. (1979). Speech as a marker of situation. In K. Scherer and H. Giles (Eds.), *Social markers in speech* (pp. 33-62). Cambridge: Cambridge University Press.

Bryden, M. (1982). *Laterality: Functional asymmetry in the intact brain.* New York: Academic Press.

Buck, R., and Duffy, R. (1980). Nonverbal communication of affect in brain-damaged patients. *Cortex, 16*, 351-362.

Cicone, M., Wapner, W., Foldi, N., Zurif, E., and Gardner, H. (1979). The relation between gesture and language in aphasic communication. *Brain and Language, 8*, 324-349.

Cicone, M., Wapner, W., and Gardner, H. (1980). Sensitivity to emotional expressions and situations in organic patients. *Cortex, 16*, 145-158.

Clark, H., and Gerrig, R. (1983). Understanding old words with new meanings. *Journal of Verbal Learning and Verbal Behavior, 22*, 591-608.

Clark, H., and Haviland, S. (1977). Comprehension and the given-new contract. In R. Freedle (Ed.), *Discourse production and comprehension* (pp. 1-40). Norwood, NJ: Ablex.

Clark, H., and Lucy, P. (1975). Understanding what is meant from what is said: A study in conversationally conveyed requests. *Journal of Verbal Learning and Verbal Behavior, 14*, 56-72.

Clark, M., and Fiske, S. (Eds.) (1982). *Affect and cognition: The seventeenth annual Carnegie symposium on cognition.* Hillsdale, NJ: Lawrence Erlbaum.

Code, C., and Müller, D. (1983). Perspectives in aphasia therapy: An overview. In C. Code and D. Müller (Eds.), *Aphasia therapy* (pp. 3-13). London: Edward Arnold.

Cohen, R., and Kelter, S. (1979). Cognitive impairment of aphasics in a colour-to-picture matching task. *Cortex, 15*, 235-245.

Cohen, R., Kelter, S., and Woll, G. (1980). Analytical competence and language impairment in aphasia. *Brain and Language, 10*, 331-347.

Collier, G. (1984). *Emotional expression.* Hillsdale, NJ: Lawrence Erlbaum.

Cummings, J., and Benson, D. (1983). *Dementia: A clinical approach.* Boston: Butterworths.

Daniloff, J., Lloyd, L., and Fristoe, M. (1983). Amer-Ind transparency. *Journal of Speech and Hearing Disorders, 48*, 103-110.

Daniloff, J., Noll, J., Fristoe, M., and Lloyd, L. (1982). Gesture recognition in patients with aphasia. *Journal of Speech and Hearing Disorders, 47*, 43-49.

Danly, M., Cooper, W., and Shapiro, B. (1983). Fundamental frequency, language processing, and linguistic structure in Wernicke's aphasia. *Brain and Language, 19*, 1-24.

Danly, M., and Shapiro, B. (1982). Speech prosody in Broca's aphasia. *Brain and Language, 16,* 171-190.

Davis, G. (1980). A critical look at PACE therapy. In R. Brookshire (Ed.), *Clinical Aphasiology Conference proceedings* (pp. 248-257). Minneapolis: BRK Publishers.

Davis, G. (1983). *A survey of adult aphasia.* Englewood Cliffs, NJ: Prentice-Hall.

Davis, G., and Holland, A. (1981). Age in understanding and treating aphasia. In D. Beasley and G. Davis (Eds.), *Aging: Communication processes and disorders* (pp. 207-228). New York: Grune and Stratton.

Davis, G., and Wilcox, M. (1981). Incorporating parameters of natural conversation in aphasia treatment. In R. Chapey (Ed.), *Language intervention strategies in adult aphasia* (pp. 169-193). Baltimore: Williams and Wilkins.

Davis, S., Artes, R., and Hoops, R. (1979). Verbal expression and expressive pantomime in aphasic patients. In Y. Lebrum and R. Hoops (Eds.), *Problems of aphasia.* Lisse, Netherlands: Swets and Zeitlinger.

Dekosky, S., Heilman, K., Bowers, D., and Valenstein, E. (1980). Recognition and discrimination of emotional faces and pictures. *Brain and Language, 9,* 206-214.

Delis, D., Foldi, N., Hamby, S., Gardner, H., and Zurif, E. (1979). A note on temporal relations between language and gestures. *Brain and Language, 8,* 350-354.

Deloche, G., and Seron, X. (1981). Sentence understanding and knowledge of the world. Evidences from a sentence-picture matching task performed by aphasic patients. *Brain and Language, 14,* 57-69.

DeRenzi, E., and Ferrari, C. (1978). The Reporter's Test: A sensitive test to detect expressive disturbances in aphasics. *Cortex, 14,* 279-293.

DeRenzi, E., Motti, F., and Nichelli, P. (1980). Imitating gestures: A quantitative approach to ideomotor apraxia. *Archives of Neurology, 37,* 6-10.

DeRenzi, E., Pieczuro, A., and Vignolo, L. (1968). Ideational apraxia: A quantitative study. *Neuropsychologia, 6,* 41-52.

DeRenzi, E., and Vignolo, L. (1962). The Token Test: A sensitive test to detect receptive disturbances in aphasia. *Brain, 85,* 665-678.

Dowden, P., Marshall, R., and Tompkins, C. (1981). Amer-Ind sign as a communicative facilitator for aphasic and apractic patients. In R. Brookshire (Ed.), *Clinical Aphasiology Conference proceedings* (pp. 133-140). Minneapolis: BRK Publishers.

Duffy, J., Keith, R., Shane, H., and Podraza, B. (1976). Performance of normal (non-brain-injured) adults on the Porch Index of Communicative Ability. In R. Brookshire (Ed.), *Clinical Aphasiology Conference proceedings* (pp. 32-42). Minneapolis: BRK Publishers.

Duffy, J., and Liles, B. (1979). A translation of Finkelnberg's (1870) lecture on aphasia as "asymbolia" with commentary. *Journal of Speech and Hearing Disorders, 44,* 156-168.

Duffy, J., and Watkins, L. (1984). The effect of response choice relatedness on pantomime and verbal recognition ability in aphasic patients. *Brain and Language, 21,* 291-306.

Duffy, R., and Buck, R. (1979). A study of the relationship between propositional (pantomime) and subpropositional (facial expression) extraverbal behaviors in aphasics. *Folia Phoniatrica, 31,* 129-136.

Duffy, R., and Duffy, J. (1981). Three studies of deficits in pantomimic expression and pantomimic recognition in aphasia. *Journal of Speech and Hearing*

Research, 24, 70-84.

Duffy, R., Duffy, J., and Mercaitis, P. (1984). Comparison of the performance of a fluent and a nonfluent aphasic on a pantomimic referential task. *Brain and Language, 21,* 260-273.

Duffy, R., Duffy, J., and Pearson, K. (1975). Pantomimic recognition in aphasics. *Journal of Speech and Hearing Research, 18,* 115-132.

Duncan, S., Jr. (1972). Some signals and rules for taking speaking turns in conversations. *Journal of Personality and Social Psychology, 23,* 283-292.

Duncan, S., Jr., and Niederehe, G. (1974). On signaling when it's your turn to speak. *Journal of Experimental Social Psychology, 10,* 234-237.

Ehrlich, K., and Rayner, K. (1983). Pronoun assignment and semantic integration during readings: Eye movements and immediacy of processing. *Journal of Verbal Learning and Verbal Behavior, 22,* 75-87.

Eisenson, J. (1984). *Adult aphasia.* Englewood Cliffs, NJ: Prentice-Hall.

Ervin-Tripp, S. (1964). An analysis of the interaction of language, topic and listener. *American Anthropologist, 66,* 86-102.

Faglioni, P., Spinnler, H., and Vignolo, L. (1969). Contrasting behavior of right and left hemisphere-damaged patients on a discriminative and a semantic task of auditory recognition. *Cortex, 5,* 366-389.

Farmer, A. (1977). Self-correctional strategies in the conversational speech of aphasic and nonaphasic brain damaged adults. *Cortex, 13,* 327-334.

Ferro, J., Martins, I., Mariano, G., and Castro-Caldas, A. (1983). CT scan correlates of gesture recognition. *Journal of Neurology, Neurosurgery, and Psychiatry, 46,* 943-952.

Ferro, J., Santos, M., Castro-Caldas, A., and Mariano, G. (1980). Gesture recognition in aphasia. *Journal of Clinical Neuropsychology, 2,* 277-292.

Feyereisen, P., and Seron, X. (1982a). Nonverbal communication and aphasia: A review. I. Comprehension. *Brain and Language, 16,* 191-212.

Feyereisen, P., and Seron, X. (1982b). Nonverbal communication and aphasia: A review. II. Expression. *Brain and Language, 16,* 213-236.

Florance, C. (1981). Methods of communication analysis used in family interaction therapy. In R. Brookshire (Ed.), *Clinical Aphasiology Conference proceedings* (pp. 204-211). Minneapolis: BRK Publishers.

Florance, C., Rabidoux, P., and McCauslin, L. (1980). An environmental manipulation approach to treating apraxia of speech. In R. Brookshire (Ed.), *Clinical Aphasiology Conference proceedings* (pp. 285-293). Minneapolis: BRK Publishers.

Flowers, C., and Danforth, L. (1979). A step-wise auditory comprehension improvement program administered to aphasic patients by family members. In R. Brookshire (Ed.), *Clinical Aphasiology Conference proceedings* (pp. 196-202). Minneapolis: BRK Publishers.

Foldi, N., Cicone, M., and Gardner, H. (1983). Pragmatic aspects of communication in brain damaged patients. In S. Segalowitz (Ed.), *Language functions and brain organization* (pp. 51-86). New York: Academic Press.

Fordyce, W., and Jones, R. (1966). The efficacy of oral and pantomime instructions for hemiplegic patients. *Archives of Physical Medicine and Rehabilitation, 46,* 676-680.

Foss, D., and Jenkins, C. (1973). Some effects of context on the comprehension of ambiguous sentences. *Journal of Verbal Learning and Verbal Behavior, 12,* 577-589.

Freedle, R. (Ed.) (1977). *Discourse production and comprehension.* Norwood, NJ: Ablex.

Freedle, R. (Ed.) (1979). *New directions in discourse processing.* Norwood, NJ: Ablex.

Freedle, R., and Duran, R. (1979). Sociolinguistic approaches to dialogue with suggested applications to cognitive science. In R. Freedle (Ed.), *New directions in discourse processing* (pp. 197-206). Norwood, NJ: Ablex.

Freedle, R., Naus, M., and Schwartz, L. (1977). Prose processing from a psychosocial perspective. In R. Freedle (Ed.), *Discourse production and comprehension* (pp. 175-192). Norwood, NJ: Ablex.

Gainotti, G. (1972). Emotional behavior and hemispheric side of lesion. *Cortex, 8,* 41-55.

Gainotti, G., and Lemmo, M. (1976). Comprehension of symbolic gestures in aphasia. *Brain and Language, 3,* 451-460.

Gallagher, T. (1977). Early discourse behavior: An analysis of children's responses to listener feedback. *Child Development, 51,* 1120-1125.

Gallagher, T., and Darnton, E. (1978). Conversational aspects of the speech of language-disordered children: Revision behaviors. *Journal of Speech and Hearing Research, 21,* 118-135.

Gandour, J., and Dardarananda, R. (1983). Identification of tonal contrasts in Thai aphasic patients. *Brain and Language, 18,* 98-114.

Gardner, H., Brownell, H., Wapner, W., and Michelow, D. (1983). Missing the point: The role of the right hemisphere in the processing of complex linguistic materials. In E. Perecman (Ed.), *Cognitive processing in the right hemisphere* (pp. 169-191). New York: Academic Press.

Gardner, H., Ling, P., Flamm, L., and Silverman, J. (1975). Comprehension and appreciation of humorous material following brain damage. *Brain, 98,* 399-412.

Gardner, H., Zurif, E., Berry T., and Baker, E. (1976). Visual communication in aphasia. *Neuropsychologia, 14,* 275-292.

Garrod, S., and Sanford, A. (1977). Interpreting anaphoric relations: The integration of semantic information while reading. *Journal of Verbal Learning and Verbal Behavior, 16,* 77-90.

Garvey, C. (1979). Contingent queries and their relations in discourse. In E. Ochs and B. Schieffelin (Eds.), *Developmental pragmatics.* New York: Academic Press.

Gibbs, R., Jr. (1981). Your wish is my command: Convention and context in interpreting indirect requests. *Journal of Verbal Learning and Verbal Behavior, 20,* 431-444.

Gibbs, R., Jr. (1982). A critical examination of the contribution of literal meaning to understanding non-literal discourse. *Text, 2,* 9-28.

Gildea, P., and Glucksberg, S. (1983). On understanding metaphor: The role of context. *Journal of Verbal Learning and Verbal Behavior, 22,* 577-590.

Giles, H., Scherer, K., and Taylor, D. (1979). Speech markers in social interaction. In K. Scherer and H. Giles (Eds.), *Social markers in speech* (pp. 343-381). Cambridge: Cambridge University Press.

Glass, A., Gazzaniga, M., and Premack, D. (1973). Artificial language training in global aphasia. *Neuropsychologia, 11,* 95-110.

Gleason, J., Goodglass, H., Green, E., Ackerman, N., and Hyde, M. (1975). The retrieval of syntax in Broca's aphasia. *Brain and Language, 2,* 451-471.

Gleason, J., Goodglass, H., Obler, L., Green, E., Hyde, M., and Weintraub, S.

(1980). Narrative strategies of aphasic and normal-speaking subjects. *Journal of Speech and Hearing Research, 23,* 370–382.

Glucksberg, S., Gildea, P., and Bookin, H. (1982). On understanding nonliteral speech: Can people ignore metaphors? *Journal of Verbal Learning and Verbal Behavior, 21,* 85–98.

Glucksberg, S., and Krauss, R. (1967). What do people say after they have learned to talk? Studies of the development of referential communication. *Merrill-Palmer Quarterly, 13,* 309–316.

Goldman-Eisler, F. (1968). *Psycholinguistics: Experiments in spontaneous speech.* New York: Academic Press.

Goodenough, C., Zurif, E., Weintraub, S., and Von Stockert, T. (1977). Aphasics' attention to grammatical morphemes. *Language and Speech, 20,* 11–19.

Goodglass, H., Blumstein, S., Gleason, J., Hyde, M., Green, E., and Statlender, S. (1979). The effect of syntactic encoding on sentence comprehension in aphasia. *Brain and Language, 7,* 201–209.

Goodglass, H., and Kaplan, E. (1963). Disturbance of gesture and pantomime in aphasia. *Brain, 86,* 703–720.

Goodglass, H., and Kaplan, E. (1972). *The assessment of aphasia and related disorders.* Philadelphia: Lea and Febiger.

Graesser, A. (1978). How to catch a fish: The memory and representation of common procedures. *Discourse Processes, 1,* 72–89.

Graves, R., Landis, T., and Goodglass, H. (1981). Laterality and sex differences for visual recognition of emotional and non-emotional words. *Neuropsychologia, 19,* 95–102.

Green, E., and Boller, F. (1974). Features of auditory comprehension in severely impaired aphasics. *Cortex, 10,* 133–145.

Greimas, A., Jacobson, R., Mayenowa, M., Saumjan, S., Steinitz, W., and Zolkiewski, S. (Eds.) (1970). *Sign, language, culture.* The Hague, Netherlands: Mouton.

Grice, H. (1975). Logic and conversation. In P. Cole and J. Morgan (Eds.), *Syntax and semantics: Speech acts* (pp. 41–58). New York: Academic Press.

Grober, E., Perecman, E., Kellar, L., and Brown, J. (1980). Lexical knowledge in anterior and posterior aphasics. *Brain and Language, 10,* 318–330.

Grossman, M. (1978). The game of the name: An examination of linguistic reference after brain damage. *Brain and Language, 6,* 112–119.

Grossman, M. (1981). A bird is a bird is a bird: Making reference within and without superordinate categories. *Brain and Language, 12,* 313–331.

Guilford, A., and O'Connor, J. (1982). Pragmatic functions in aphasia. *Journal of Communication Disorders, 15,* 337–346.

Gurland, G., Chwat, S., and Wollner, S. (1982). Establishing a communication profile in adult aphasia: Analysis of communicative acts and conversational sequences. In R. Brookshire (Ed.), *Clinical Aphasiology Conference proceedings* (pp. 18–27). Minneapolis: BRK Publishers.

Haberlandt, K., and Bingham, G. (1978). Verbs contribute to the coherence of brief narratives: Reading related and unrelated sentence triplets. *Journal of Verbal Learning and Verbal Behavior, 17,* 419–425.

Halliday, M. (1975). *Learning how to mean: Explorations in the development of language.* New York: Elsevier.

Harris, D., and Vanderheiden, G. (1980). Augmentative communication techniques. In R. Schiefelbusch (Ed.), *Nonspeech language and communication: Analysis and intervention* (pp. 259–301). Baltimore: University Park Press.

Harrison, R. (1974). *Beyond words: An introduction to nonverbal communication.* Englewood Cliffs, NJ: Prentice-Hall.

Haviland, S., and Clark, H. (1974). What's new? Acquiring new information as a process in comprehension. *Journal of Verbal Learning and Verbal Behavior, 13,* 512–521.

Heeschen, C. (1980). Strategies of decoding actor-object relations by aphasic patients. *Cortex, 16,* 5–19.

Heilman, K. (1973). Ideational apraxia—a re-definition. *Brain, 96,* 861–864.

Heilman, K., Bowers, D., Speedie, L., and Coslett, H. (1984). Comprehension of affective and nonaffective prosody. *Neurology, 34,* 917–921.

Heilman, K., and Scholes, R. (1976). The nature of comprehension errors in Broca's, conduction and Wernicke's aphasics. *Cortex, 12,* 258–265.

Heilman, K., Scholes, R., and Watson, R. (1975). Auditory affective agnosia: Disturbed comprehension of affective speech. *Journal of Neurology, Neurosurgery, and Psychiatry, 38,* 69–72.

Heilman, K., Schwartz, H., and Watson, R. (1978). Hypoarousal in patients with the neglect syndrome and emotional indifference. *Neurology, 28,* 229–232.

Helm, N., and Barresi, B. (1980). Voluntary control of involuntary utterances: A treatment approach for severe aphasia. In R. Brookshire (Ed.), *Clinical Aphasiology Conference proceedings* (pp. 308–315). Minneapolis: BRK Publishers.

Helm-Estabrooks, N., Fitzpatrick, P., and Barresi, B. (1981). Response of an agrammatic patient to a syntax stimulation program for aphasia. *Journal of Speech and Hearing Disorders, 46,* 422–427.

Helm-Estabrooks, N., Fitzpatrick, P., and Barresi, B. (1982). Visual action therapy for global aphasia. *Journal of Speech and Hearing Disorders, 47,* 385–389.

Hirst, W., and Brill, G. (1980). Contextual aspects of pronoun assignment. *Journal of Verbal Learning and Verbal Behavior, 19,* 168–175.

Hirst, W., LeDoux, J., and Stein, S. (1984). Constraints on the processing of indirect speech acts: Evidence from aphasiology. *Brain and Language, 23,* 26–33.

Holland, A. (1975, November). *Aphasics as communicators: A model and its implications.* Paper presented to the American Speech-Language-Hearing Association, Washington, DC.

Holland, A. (1977). Some practical considerations in aphasia rehabilitation. In M. Sullivan and M.S. Kommers (Eds.), *Rationale for adult aphasia therapy* (pp. 167–180). University of Nebraska Medical Center, Lincoln.

Holland, A. (1978). Functional communication in the treatment of aphasia. In L.J. Bradford (Ed.), *Communicative Disorders: An audio journal for continuing education.* New York: Grune and Stratton.

Holland, A. (1980). *Communicative abilities in daily living.* Baltimore: University Park Press.

Holland, A. (1982). Observing functional communication of aphasic adults. *Journal of Speech and Hearing Disorders, 47,* 50–56.

Holland, A., and Sonderman, J. (1974). Effects of a program based on the Token Test for teaching comprehension skills to aphasics. *Journal of Speech and Hearing Research, 17,* 589–598.

Houghton, P., Pettit, J., and Towey, M. (1982). Measuring communication competence in global aphasia. In R. Brookshire (Ed.), *Clinical Aphasiology Conference proceedings* (pp. 28–39). Minneapolis: BRK Publishers.

Huber, W., and Gleber, J. (1982). Linguistic and nonlinguistic processing of narratives in aphasia. *Brain and Language, 16,* 1–18.

Irwin, D., Bock, J., and Stanovich, K. (1982). Effects of information structure cues on visual word processing. *Journal of Verbal Learning and Verbal Behavior, 21*, 307-325.

Jaffe, J. (1978). Parliamentary procedure and the brain. In A. Seigman and S. Feldstein (Eds.), *Nonverbal behavior and communication* (pp. 55-66). Hillsdale, NJ: Lawrence Erlbaum.

Kearns, K., Simmons, N., and Sisterhen, C. (1982). Gestural sign (Amer-Ind) as a facilitator of verbalization in patients with aphasia. In R. Brookshire (Ed.), *Clinical Aphasiology Conference proceedings* (pp. 183-191). Minneapolis: BRK Publishers.

Keith, R. (1972). *Speech and language rehabilitation: A workbook for the neurologically impaired.* Danville, IL: Interstate Printers and Publishers.

Kelter, S., Cohen, R., Engel, D., List, G., and Strohner, H. (1977). The conceptual structure of aphasic and schizophrenic patients in a nonverbal sorting task. *Journal of Psycholinguistic Research, 6*, 279-303.

Kennedy, J. (1983). Treatment of Wernicke's aphasia. In W.H. Perkins (Ed.), *Language Handicaps in Adults* (pp. 15-24). New York: Thieme-Stratton.

Kertesz, A., and McCabe, P. (1977). Recovery patterns and prognosis in aphasia. *Brain, 100*, 1-18.

Kieras, D. (1978). Good and bad structure in simple paragraphs: Effects on apparent theme, reading time, and recall. *Journal of Verbal Learning and Verbal Behavior, 17*, 13-28.

Kimbarow, M. (1982, November). Discourse analysis: A look at clinicians' conversational strategies in treatment. Paper presented at the Annual Meeting of the American Speech-Language-Hearing Association, Toronto.

Kimbarow, M., and Brookshire, R. (1983). The influence of communicative context on aphasic speakers' use of pronouns. In R. Brookshire (Ed.), *Clinical Aphasiology Conference proceedings* (pp. 195-201). Minneapolis: BRK Publishers.

Kintsch, W. (1977). On comprehending stories. In M. Just and P. Carpenter (Eds.), *Cognitive processes in comprehension* (pp. 33-62). Hillsdale, NJ: Lawrence Erlbaum.

Kintsch, W., and van Dijk, T. (1978). Toward a model of text comprehension and production. *Psychological Review, 85*, 363-394.

Krauss, R., and Weinheimer, S. (1964). Changes in reference phrases as a function of frequency of usage in social interaction: A preliminary study. *Psychonomic Science, 1*, 113-114.

Kreindler, A., Gheorghita, N., and Voinescu, I. (1971). Analysis of verbal reception of a complex order with three elements in aphasics. *Brain, 94*, 375-386.

Kudo, T. (1984). The effect of semantic plausibility on sentence comprehension in aphasia. *Brain and Language, 21*, 208-218.

Larkins, P., and Webster, E. (1981). The use of gestures in dyads consisting of an aphasic and nonaphasic adult. In R. Brookshire (Ed.), *Clinical Aphasiology Conference proceedings* (pp. 120-127). Minneapolis: BRK Publishers.

Laver, J., and Trudgill, P. (1979). Phonetic and linguistic markers in speech. In K. Scherer and H. Giles (Eds.), *Social markers in speech* (pp. 1-32). Cambridge: Cambridge University Press.

LeDoux, J., Blum, C., and Hirst, W. (1983). Inferential processing of context: Studies of cognitively impaired subjects. *Brain and Language, 19*, 216-224.

Lesser, R. (1979). Turning tokens into things: Linguistic and mnestic aspects of the initial sections of the Token Test. In F. Boller and M. Dennis (Eds.), *Auditory comprehension: Clinical and experimental studies with the Token Test* (pp. 71–85). New York: Academic Press.

Levin, S., and Koch-Weser, M. (1982). Right hemispheric superiority in the recognition of famous faces. *Brain and Cognition, 1,* 10–22.

Levy, J., Trevarthen, C., and Sperry R. (1972). Perception of bilateral chimeric figures following hemisphere disconnexion. *Brain, 95,* 61–68.

Ley R., and Bryden, M. (1979). Hemispheric differences in processing emotions and faces. *Brain and Language, 7,* 127–138.

Lieberman, P. (1967). *Intonation, perception, and language.* Cambridge, MA: MIT Press.

Linebaugh, C., Kryzer, K., Oden, S., and Myers, P. (1982). Reapportionment of communicative burden in aphasia: A study of narrative instructions. In R. Brookshire (Ed.), *Clinical Aphasiology Conference proceedings* (pp. 4–9). Minneapolis: BRK Publishers.

Lohmann, L., and Prescott, T. (1978). The effects of substituting "objects" for "forms" on the Revised Token Test (RTT) performance of aphasic subjects. In R. Brookshire (Ed.), *Clinical Aphasiology Conference proceedings* (pp. 138–146). Minneapolis: BRK Publishers.

Lubinski, R. (1981a). Environmental language intervention. In R. Chapey (Ed.), *Language intervention strategies in adult aphasia* (pp. 223–245). Baltimore: Williams and Wilkins.

Lubinski, R. (1981b). Speech, language, and audiology programs in home and health care agencies and nursing homes. In D.S. Beasley and G.A. Davis (Eds.), *Aging: Communication processes and disorders* (pp. 339–356). New York: Grune and Stratton.

Lubinski, R., Duchan, J., and Weitzner-Lin, B. (1980). Analysis of breakdowns and repairs in aphasic adult communication. In R. Brookshire (Ed.), *Clinical Aphasiology Conference proceedings* (pp. 111–116). Minneapolis: BRK Publishers.

MacWhinney, B., and Bates, E. (1978). Sentential devices for conveying givenness and newness: A cross-cultural developmental study. *Journal of Verbal Learning and Verbal Behavior, 17,* 539–558.

Mandler, J., and Johnson, N. (1977). Remembrance of things parsed: Story structure and recall. *Cognitive Psychology, 9,* 111–151.

Markel, N., Phillis, J., Vargas, R., and Howard, K. (1972). Personality traits associated with voice types. *Journal of Psycholinguistic Research, 1,* 249–255.

Marshall, R. (1976). Word retrieval behavior of aphasic adults. *Journal of Speech and Hearing Disorders, 41,* 444–451.

Marshall, R., and Tompkins, C. (1981). Identifying behavior associated with verbal self-corrections of aphasic clients. *Journal of Speech and Hearing Disorders, 46,* 168–173.

Marshall, R., and Tompkins, C. (1982). Verbal self-correction behaviors of fluent and nonfluent aphasic subjects. *Brain and Language, 15,* 292-306.

Martino, A., Pizzamiglio, L., and Razzano, C. (1976). A new version of the "Token Test" for aphasics: A concrete objects form. *Journal of Communication Disorders, 9,* 1–5.

Martinoff, J., Martinoff, R., and Stokke, V. (1980). *Language rehabilitation: Auditory comprehension.* Tigard, OR: C.C. Publications.

McDonald, E. (1980). Early identification and treatment of children at risk for speech development. In R. Schiefelbusch (Ed.), *Nonspeech language and communication: Analysis and intervention* (pp. 49–79). Baltimore: University Park Press.

Morgan, J. (1979). Observations on the pragmatics of metaphor. In A. Ortony (Ed.), *Metaphor and thought* (pp. 136–147). Cambridge: Cambridge University Press.

Morrow, L., Vrtunski, P., Kim, Y., and Boller, F. (1981). Arousal responses to emotional stimuli and laterality of lesion. *Neuropsychologia, 19,* 65–71.

Newhoff, M., Bugbee, J., and Ferreira, A. (1981). A change of PACE: Spouses as treatment targets. In R. Brookshire (Ed.), *Clinical Aphasiology Conference proceedings* (pp. 234–243). Minneapolis: BRK Publishers.

Newhoff, M., Tonkovich, J., Schwartz, S., and Burgess, E. (1982). Revision strategies in aphasia. In R. Brookshire (Ed.), *Clinical Aphasiology Conference proceedings* (pp. 83–84). Minneapolis: BRK Publishers.

Nicholas, L., and Brookshire, R. (1983). Syntactic simplification and context: Effects on sentence comprehension by aphasic adults. In R. Brookshire (Ed.), *Clinical Aphasiology Conference proceedings* (pp. 166–172). Minneapolis: BRK Publishers.

Orazi, D., and Wilcox, M. (1982, November). The modification of spontaneous speech in language-disordered children. Paper presented to the annual meeting of the American Speech-Language-Hearing Association, Toronto.

Ortony, A., Reynolds, R., and Arter, J. (1978). Metaphor: Theoretical and empirical research. *Psychological Bulletin, 85,* 919–943.

Ortony, A., Schallert, D., Reynolds, R., and Antos, S. (1978). Interpreting metaphors and idioms: Some effects of context on comprehension. *Journal of Verbal Learning and Verbal Behavior, 17,* 465–477.

Owens, R., and House, L. (1984). Decision-making processes in augmentative communication. *Journal of Speech and Hearing Disorders, 49,* 18–25.

Paivio, A. (1979). Psychological processes in the comprehension of metaphor. In A. Ortony (Ed.), *Metaphor and thought* (pp. 150–171). Cambridge: Cambridge University Press.

Pashek, G., and Brookshire, R. (1982). Effects of rate of speech and linguistic stress on auditory paragraph comprehension of aphasic individuals. *Journal of Speech and Hearing Research, 25,* 377–382.

Peterson, L., and Kirshner, H. (1981). Gestural impairment and gestural ability in aphasia: A review. *Brain and Language, 14,* 333–348.

Pierce, R., and Beekman, L. (1983). Effects of linguistic and extralinguistic context on semantic and syntactic processing in aphasia. In R. Brookshire (Ed.), *Clinical Aphasiology Conference proceedings* (pp. 173–176). Minneapolis: BRK Publishers.

Porch, B. (1967). *Porch index of communicative ability: Vol. I. Theory and development.* Palo Alto, CA: Consulting Psychologists Press.

Porch, B. (1981). *Porch index of communicative ability: Vol. II. Administration, scoring, and interpretation* (3rd ed.). Palo Alto, CA: Consulting Psychologists Press.

Prinz, P. (1980). A note on requesting strategies in adult aphasics. *Journal of Communication Disorders, 13,* 65–73.

Prinz, P., Snow, C., and Wagenaar, E. (1978). Recovery from aphasia: Spontaneous speech versus language comprehension. *Brain and Language, 6,* 192–211.

Prutting, C. (1982). Pragmatics as social competence. *Journal of Speech and Hearing Disorders, 47,* 123–133.

Prutting, C., and Kirchner, D. (1983). Applied pragmatics. In T. Gallagher and C. Prutting (Eds.), *Pragmatic assessment and intervention issues in language* (pp. 29–64). San Diego: College-Hill Press.

Rao, P., and Horner, J. (1978). Gesture as a deblocking modality in a severe aphasic patient. In R. Brookshire (Ed.), *Clinical Aphasiology Conference proceedings* (pp. 180–187). Minneapolis: BRK Publishers.

Rees, N. (1978). Pragmatics of language: Applications to normal and disordered language development. In R. Schiefelbusch (Ed.), *Bases of language intervention* (pp. 191–268). Baltimore: University Park Press.

Rees, N. (1982). An overview of pragmatics, or what is in the box? In J. Irwin (Ed.), *Pragmatics: The role in language development* (pp. 1–13). LaVerne, CA: Fox Point Publishers.

Richards, I. (1936). *The philosophy of rhetoric.* London: Oxford University Press.

Ripich, D., Terrell, B., and Spinelli, F. (1983). Discourse cohesion in senile dementia of the Alzheimer type. In R. Brookshire (Ed.), *Clinical Aphasiology Conference proceedings* (pp. 316–321). Minneapolis: BRK Publishers.

Ritter, E. (1976a). Modular therapy: A practical approach to life situations. In R. Brookshire (Ed.), *Clinical Aphasiology Conference proceedings* (pp. 200–203). Minneapolis: BRK Publishers.

Ritter, E. (1976b). Effects of environmental stimulation upon the language output of aphasic patients. In R. Brookshire (Ed.), *Clinical Aphasiology Conference proceedings* (pp. 278–290). Minneapolis: BRK Publishers.

Rivers, D., and Love, R. (1980). Language performance on visual processing tasks in right hemisphere lesion cases. *Brain and Language, 10,* 348–366.

Robinson, R., and Benson, D. (1981). Depression in aphasic patients: Frequency, severity, and clinical-pathological correlations. *Brain and Language, 14,* 282–291.

Robinson, W. (1972). *Language and social behavior.* Baltimore: Penguin.

Rosch, E. (1977). Style variables in referential language: A study of social class difference and its effect on dyadic communication. In R. Freedle (Ed.), *Discourse production and comprehension* (pp. 141–159). Norwood, NJ: Ablex.

Rosenbek, J. (1979). Wrinkled feet. In R. Brookshire (Ed.), *Clinical Aphasiology Conference proceedings* (pp. 163–176). Minneapolis: BRK Publishers.

Rosenbek, J. (1983). Some challenges for clinical aphasiologists. In J. Milles, D.E. Yoder, and R. Schiefelbusch (Eds.), *Contemporary issues in language intervention* (pp. 317–325). Rockville, MD: American Speech-Language-Hearing Association.

Rosenfeld, H. (1978). Conversational control functions of nonverbal behavior. In A. Siegman and S. Feldstein (Eds.), *Nonverbal behavior and communication* (pp. 291–328). New York: John Wiley and Sons.

Ross, E. (1981). The aprosodias: Functional-anatomic organization of the affective components of language in the right hemisphere. *Archives of Neurology, 38,* 561–569.

Roth, F., and Spekman, N. (1984). Assessing the pragmatic abilities of children: Part 1. Organizational framework and assessment parameters. *Journal of Speech and Hearing Disorders, 49,* 2–11.

Sacks, H., Schegloff, E., and Jefferson, G. (1974). A simplest systematics for the organization of turn-taking for conversation. *Language, 50,* 606–735.

Samuels, S., and Eisenberg, P. (1981). A framework for understanding the reading process. In F. Pirozzolo and M. Wittrock (Eds.), *Neuropsychological and cognitive processes in reading.* New York: Academic Press.

Sarno, M. (1969). *The Functional communication profile: Manual of directions.*

New York: New York University Medical Center—The Institute of Rehabilitation Medicine.

Sarno, M., and Levita, E. (1981). Some observations on the nature of recovery in global aphasia after stroke. *Journal of Brain and Language, 13,* 1–12.

Schank, R., and Abelson, R. (1977). *Scripts, plans, goals, and understanding.* Hillsdale, NJ: Lawrence Erlbaum.

Scherer, K. (1979). Personality markers in speech. In K. Scherer and H. Giles (Eds.), *Social markers in speech.* Cambridge: Cambridge University Press.

Schienberg, S., and Holland, A. (1980). Conversational turn-taking in Wernicke's aphasia. In R. Brookshire (Ed.), *Clinical Aphasiology Conference proceedings* (pp. 106–110). Minneapolis: BRK Publishers.

Schlanger, B., Schlanger, P., and Gerstman, L. (1976). The perception of emotionally toned sentences by right hemisphere-damaged and aphasic subjects. *Brain and Language, 3,* 396–403.

Schlanger, P. (1978). *Picture communication cards.* Tucson, AZ: Communication Skill Builders.

Schlanger, P. (1980). *What's the solut on?* Tucson, AZ: Communication Skill Builders.

Schlanger, P., and Schlanger, B. (1970). Adapting role playing activities with aphasic patients. *Journal of Speech and Hearing Disorders, 35,* 229–235.

Searle, J. (1969). *Speech acts: An essay in the philosophy of language.* London: Cambridge University Press.

Searle, J. (1979). Metaphor. In A. Ortony (Ed.), *Metaphor and thought* (pp. 92–123). Cambridge: Cambridge University Press.

Semenza, C., Denes, G., Lucchese, D., and Bisiacchi, P. (1980). Selective deficit of conceptual structures in aphasia: Class versus thematic relations. *Brain and Language, 10,* 243–248.

Seron, X., and Deloche, G. (1981). Processing of locatives "in," "on," and "under" by aphasic patients: An analysis of the regression hypothesis. *Brain and Language, 14,* 70–80.

Seron, X., Van Der Kaa, M., Remitz, A., and Van Der Linden, M. (1979). Pantomime interpretation and aphasia. *Neuropsychologia, 17,* 661–668.

Seron, X., Van Der Kaa, M., Van Der Linden, M., Remitz, A., and Feyereisen, P. (1982). Decoding paralinguistic signals: Effect of semantic and prosodic cues on aphasics' comprehension. *Journal of Communication Disorders, 15,* 223–231.

Sies, L., and Butler, R. (1963). A personal account of dysphasia. *Journal of Speech and Hearing Disorders, 28,* 261–266.

Silverman, F. (1980). *Communication for the speechless.* Englewood Cliffs, NJ: Prentice-Hall.

Simmons, N., and Zorthian, A. (1979). Use of symbolic gestures in a case of fluent aphasia. In R. Brookshire (Ed.), *Clinical Aphasiology Conference proceedings* (pp. 278–285). Minneapolis: BRK Publishers.

Skelly, M. (1979). *Amer-Ind gestural code based on universal American Indian hand talk.* New York: Elsevier.

Smith, B., Brown, B., Strong, W., and Rencher, A. (1975). Effects of speech rate on personality perception. *Language and Speech, 18,* 145–152.

Sowa, J. (1983). *Conceptual structures: Information processing in mind and machine.* Reading, MA: Addison-Wesley.

Sparks, R. (1978). Parastandardized examination guidelines for adult aphasia. *British Journal of Disorders of Communication, 13,* 135–146.

Spiegel, D., Jones, L., and Wepman, J. (1965). Test responses as predictors of free-speech characteristics in aphasic patients. *Journal of Speech and Hearing Research, 8,* 349–362.

Spinnler, H., and Vignolo, L. (1966). Impaired recognition of meaningful sounds in aphasia. *Cortex, 2,* 337–348.

Spradlin, J., and Siegel, G. (1982). Language training in natural and clinical environments. *Journal of Speech and Hearing Disorders, 47,* 2–6.

Stachowiak, F., Huber, W., Poeck, K., and Kerschensteiner, M. (1977). Text comprehension in aphasia. *Brain and Language, 4,* 177–195.

Swinney, D. (1979). Lexical access during sentence comprehension: (Re)Consideration of context effects. *Journal of Verbal Learning and Verbal Behavior, 18,* 645–660.

Swinney, D., and Cutler, A. (1979). The access and processing of idiomatic expressions. *Journal of Verbal Learning and Verbal Behavior, 18,* 523–534.

Tanner, D. (1980). Loss and grief: Implication for the speech-language pathologist and audiologist. *Asha, 22,* 916–928.

Taylor, M. (1965). A measurement of functional communication in aphasia. *Archives of Physical Medicine and Rehabilitation, 46,* 101–107.

Thorndyke, P. (1977). Cognitive structures in comprehension and memory of narrative discourse. *Cognitive Psychology, 9,* 77–110.

Tonkovich, J., and Loverso, F. (1982). A training matrix approach for gestural acquisition by the agrammatic patient. In R. Brookshire (Ed.), *Clinical Aphasiology Conference proceedings* (pp. 283–288). Minneapolis: BRK Publishers.

Towey, M., and Pettit, J. (1980). Improving communication competence in global aphasia. In R. Brookshire (Ed.), *Clinical Aphasiology Conference proceedings* (pp. 139–146). Minneapolis: BRK Publishers.

Tucker, D., Watson, R., and Heilman, K. (1977). Discrimination and evocation of affectively intoned speech in patients with right parietal disease. *Neurology, 27,* 947–950.

Tyler, S., and Voss, J. (1982). Attitude and knowledge effects in prose processing. *Journal of Verbal Learning and Verbal Behavior, 21,* 524–538.

Ulatowska, H., Doyel, A., Stern, R., Haynes, S., and North, A. (1983). Production of procedural discourse in aphasia. *Brain and Language, 18,* 315–341.

Ulatowska, H., Freedman-Stern, R., Doyel, A., Macaluso-Haynes, S., and North, A. (1983). Production of narrative discourse in aphasia. *Brain and Language, 19,* 317–334.

Ulatowska, H., Haynes, S., Hildebrand, B., and Richardson, S. (1977). The aphasic individual: A speaker and a listener, not a patient. In R. Brookshire (Ed.), *Clinical Aphasiology Conference proceedings* (pp. 198–213). Minneapolis: BRK Publishers.

Ulatowska, H., Macaluso-Haynes, S., and Mendel-Richardson, S. (1976). The assessment of communicative competence in aphasia. In R. Brookshire (Ed.), *Clinical Aphasiology Conference proceedings* (pp. 22–31). Minneapolis: BRK Publishers.

Ulatowska, H., North, A., and Macaluso-Haynes, S. (1981). Production of narrative and procedural discourse in aphasia. *Brain and Language, 13,* 345–371.

van Dijk, T. (1977). Semantic macro-structures and knowledge frames in discourse comprehension. In M. Just and P. Carpenter (Eds.), *Cognitive processes in comprehension* (pp. 3–32). Hillsdale, NJ: Lawrence Erlbaum.

van Dijk, T., and Kintsch, W. (1983). *Strategies of discourse comprehension.* New York: Academic Press.

Varney, N. (1978). Linguistic correlates of pantomime recognition in aphasic patients. *Journal of Neurology, Neurosurgery, and Psychiatry, 41,* 546–568.

Varney, N. (1982). Pantomime recognition defect in aphasia: Implications for the concept of asymbolia. *Brain and Language, 15,* 32–39.

Varney, N., and Benton, A. (1982). Qualitative aspects of pantomime recognition defect in aphasia. *Brain and Cognition, 1,* 132–139.

Waller, M., and Darley, F. (1978). The influence of context on the auditory comprehension of paragraphs by aphasic subjects. *Journal of Speech and Hearing Research, 21,* 732–745.

Wapner, W., Hamby, S., and Gardner, H. (1981). The role of the right hemisphere in the apprehension of complex linguistic materials. *Brain and Language, 14,* 15–33.

Warren, R., and Datta, K. (1981). The return of speech 4½ years post head injury: A case report. In R. Brookshire (Ed.), *Clinical Aphasiology Conference proceedings* (pp. 301–308). Minneapolis: BRK Publishers.

Weaver, R. (1967). *A rhetoric and composition handbook.* New York: William Morrow.

Webster, E., and Newhoff, M. (1981). Intervention with families of communicatively impaired adults. In D. Beasley and A. Davis (Eds.), *Aging: Communication processes and disorders* (pp. 229–240). New York: Grune and Stratton.

Wegner, M., Brookshire R., and Nicholas, L. (1984). Comprehension of main ideas and details in coherent and noncoherent discourse by aphasic and nonaphasic listeners. *Brain and Language, 21,* 37–51.

Weiner, S., and Goodenough, D. (1977). A move toward a psychology of conversation. In R. Freedle (Ed.), *Discourse production and comprehension* (pp. 213–225). Norwood, NJ: Ablex.

Wepman, J. (1972). Aphasia therapy: A new look. *Journal of Speech and Hearing Disorders, 37,* 203–214.

Wepman, J. (1976). Aphasia: Language without thought or thought without language. *Asha, 18,* 131–136.

Wiig, E. (1982). *Let's talk: Developing prosocial communication skills.* Columbus, OH: Charles E. Merrill.

Wilcox, M. (1984). Developmental language disorders: Preschoolers. In A. Holland (Ed.), *Language disorders in children* (pp. 101–128). San Diego: College-Hill Press.

Wilcox, M., and Davis, G. (1977). Speech act analysis of aphasic communication in individual and group settings. In R. Brookshire (Ed.), *Clinical Aphasiology Conference proceedings* (pp. 166–174). Minneapolis: BRK Publishers.

Wilcox, M., and Davis, G. (1978, November). *Promoting aphasic communicative effectiveness.* Paper presented to the American Speech-Language-Hearing Association, San Francisco.

Wilcox, M., and Davis, G. (1979, November). *Promoting aphasic communicative effectiveness.* Videotape presented to the annual meeting of the American Speech-Language-Hearing Association, Atlanta.

Wilcox, M., Davis, G., and Leonard, L. (1978). Aphasics' comprehension of contextually conveyed meaning. *Brain and Language, 6,* 362–377.

Wilcox, M., and Leonard, L. (1978). The experimental acquisition of Wh questions in language-disoriented children. *Journal of Speech and Hearing Research, 21,* 220–239.

Wilcox, M., and Webster, E. (1980). Early discourse behavior: An analysis of children's responses to listener feedback. *Child Development, 51,* 1120–1125.

Williams, C., and Stevens, K. (1972). Emotions and speech: Some acoustical correlates. *Journal of the Acoustical Society of America, 52,* 1238-1250.

Winograd, T. (1977). A framework for understanding discourse. In M. Just and P. Carpenter (Eds.), *Cognitive processes in comprehension.* Hillsdale, NJ: Lawrence Erlbaum.

Winner, E., and Gardner, H. (1977). Comprehension of metaphor in brain damaged patients. *Brain, 100,* 717-729.

Wollner, S., and Geller, E. (1982). Methods of assessing pragmatic abilities. In J. Irwin (Ed.), *Pragmatics: The role in language development* (pp. 135-160). LaVerne, CA: Fox Point Publishing.

Yorkston, K., and Beukelman, D. (1980). An analysis of connected speech samples of aphasic and normal speakers. *Journal of Speech and Hearing Disorders, 45,* 27-36.

Yorkston, K., Beukelman, D., and Flowers, C. (1980). Efficiency of information exchange between aphasic speakers and their communication partners. In R. Brookshire (Ed.), *Clinical Aphasiology Conference proceedings* (pp. 96-105). Minneapolis: BRK Publishers.

Zurif, E. (1980). Language mechanisms: A neuropsychological perspective. *American Scientist, 68,* 305-3111.

Author Index

A

Abelson, R., 7
Ackerman, N., 28
Antos, S., 23
Apel, K., 50, 78
Archer, L., 145
Arter, J., 22, 24
Artes, R., 47

B

Baker, E., 145
Bandura, A., 93
Barnes, G., 7
Barresi, B., 46, 67, 134
Basso, A., 34
Bates, E., 19
Baum, S., 33, 64
Bear, D., 32
Beekman, L., 27, 30, 35
Benson, D., 38, 39
Benton, A., 44
Bern, H., 5
Berndt, R., 26
Berry, T., 145
Berry, W., 146
Beukelman, D., 26, 40, 45, 143
Biber, C., 27
Bingham, G., 6
Bisiacchi, P., 37
Black, J., 5
Bliss, L., 143
Blum, C., 27
Blumstein, S., 27, 33
Bock, J., 5
Boller, F., 32, 39, 40, 64
Bond, S., 31, 85
Bookin, H., 24

Bowers, D., 32, 38
Brill, G., 4, 27
Britton, B., 12
Brookshire, R., 28, 29, 30, 33, 51, 59, 64, 113, 123, 125
Brown, B., 8
Brown, J., 37
Brown, P., 9, 10, 13
Brownell, H., 29
Browning-Hall, J., 50
Bryden, M., 32, 38, 39, 42
Buck, R., 39, 43, 47, 48, 51
Bugbee, J., 149
Burgess, E., 51
Butler, R., 125

C

Carmazza, A., 26, 37
Castro-Caldas, A., 43, 44
Chwat, S., 40
Cicone, M., 26, 34, 35, 38, 40, 41, 42, 48
Clark, H., 1, 15, 18, 21, 23
Clark, M., 8
Code, C., 122
Cohen, R., 34, 35, 37
Cole, M., 40
Collier, G., 8
Cooper, W., 32
Coslett, H., 32
Culter, A., 23
Cummings, J., 38

D

Danforth, L., 131
Daniloff, J., 33, 44, 45, 135
Daniloff, R., 33

Subject Index